M000265745

Functional Phonetics Workbook

Second Edition

Keon McKay

Functional Phonetics Workbook

Second Edition

Mary Lou Marsoun Cancio, M.A., CCC-SLP
Sadanand Singh, Ph.D.

Contributions by
Sara Snell, B.A.

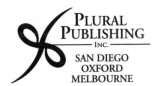

PLURAL
PUBLISHING
INC.
SAN DIEGO
OXFORD
MELBOURNE

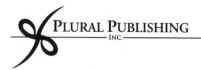

5521 Ruffin Road
San Diego, CA 92123

e-mail: info@pluralpublishing.com
Web site: http://www.pluralpublishing.com

Typeset in 11/14 Stone Informal by Flanagan's Publishing Services, Inc.
Printed in the United States of America by McNaughton and Gunn, Inc.
17 16 15   2 3 4 5

ISBN-13: 978-1-59756-990-3
ISBN-10: 1-59756-990-9

Keon McKay

Contents

Preface

The *Functional Phonetics Workbook* was designed to be used in several ways. It is a valuable classroom resource for instructors who teach an introductory phonetics course. It can be used, with the accompanying CDs, for individuals to learn the International Phonetic Alphabet (IPA) who may not have access to formal instruction. The *Workbook* also provides a convenient review format for those who require a review of their phonetic transcription skills. For example, a first-semester clinician who has not reviewed phonetics since taking the introductory course during their first semester of communicative disorders courses. The student may find it helpful to review if they have been assigned an articulation or phonological process disorder client.

The *Workbook* focuses on the basics of phonetic transcription in Standard American English, which makes it a very valuable resource for individuals who are learning to speak English. Students should find the Study Cards a very helpful study tool for learning the IPA sound/symbol association. All of these cards can now be listened to on CD 3. Each track corresponds to the study card number.

New material which provides more information on the concepts of syllables, word stress and central vowels has been added to the second edition. In addition, Study Questions have been included after each chapter. However, this text remains a helpful resource for mastering basic use of the IPA. Having taught an introductory Phonetics course since 1994 has refined my view of the basics required for students to become competent transcribers. The success of hundreds of my students as they become proficient using the IPA has brought great satisfaction. May you experience the same success and enjoy the learning process.

Mary Lou Marsoun Cancio,
M.A., CCC-SLP

Acknowledgments

The second edition of this text is dedicated to the memory of Dr. Sadanand Singh. I was honored to serve as his co-author for the first edition. His passing has left a void in our hearts and the profession of speech-language pathology.

As mentioned in the first edition, my gratitude to Dr. Thayne Hedges who instilled my love of Phonetics when he taught the course. Thanks to Sara for her suggestions and hard work.

To the wonderful group at Plural Publishing—my thanks to you.

As with the first edition, the generosity of Pamela Wing and innovative page format of Cheryl Andrews is appreciated.

The original recordings by Kimberly Lenz, Andrew Sessions, Scott Calderwood, and Kevin Wing continue to sound professional. In addition, many thanks to Taylor Harris who recorded for the first edition and graciously agreed to do more recording for the second edition. Continued thanks to Ericka Olsen, Kim Bettencourt, and Pamela Wing, who listened to the CD recordings for interlistener reliability.

Thanks again to Ray Settle and Eric Sherbon of Maximus Studios in Fresno, California for making the recording process a smooth one.

And love to all the Marsouns and my friends who continue to be a blessing.

Mary Lou Marsoun Cancio

Workbook Format

For each phoneme, an exercise to help you determine initial-medial-final phoneme position is provided, including the transcription exercise number and corresponding CD track. Remember that not all of the words in these exercises contain the specified phoneme. The goal is to ensure the student is not confused by spelling and focus on listening to the *sound* of the phonemes in the word.

Each track is also identified by the CD number (1, 2 or 3). A phonetic transcription exercise follows, with a reference to the Phoneme Study Card and CD track.

A phoneme description page is provided for IPA phonemes. Each page is organized to provide the following information (see example on next page): (1) description of place and manner and listing of distinctive features, (2) vocal fold and velopharyngeal port position, (3) tongue position and how the phoneme is produced, (4) variations in spelling, (5) word position in Standard American English (SAE), and (6) clinical information. The Clinical Information section includes a listing of a consonant cognate (sound made in the same place and the same manner), common articulatory substitutions (replacement of one phoneme for another), or omission (absence of a phoneme and another phoneme does not replace it).

A Crossword Puzzle and Word Search are also included and provide more practice in phonetic transcription. Answers to all of the Crossword Puzzles and Word Searches are listed in Appendix B: Answers to Exercises.

Example of the Phoneme Description Page

Distinctive Features	Tongue Position
1.	3.
Voicing/Velopharyngeal Port	**Spelling Variations**
2.	4.
Word Position	**Clinical Information**
5.	6.

CHAPTER

1

The International Phonetic Alphabet (IPA)

Learning Objectives

After reading this chapter, you will be able to:

1. State why the International Phonetic Alphabet (IPA) was developed.

2. Name and explain three reference points for studying speech sounds.

3. Define Phonetics and explain why it is a functional tool.

4. Identify the origin of many of the symbols of the IPA.

The English have no respect for their language, and will not teach their children to speak it. They cannot spell it because they have nothing to spell it with but an old foreign alphabet of which only the consonants—and not all of them—have any agreed speech value. Consequently no man can teach himself what it should sound like from reading it . . .

George Bernard Shaw, Preface to *Pygmalion*

As George Bernard Shaw laments, the "old foreign alphabet" does not provide a reliable sound-symbol representation of speech sounds.

In 1886, the International Phonetic Association developed a sound-symbol system based on an earlier alphabet developed by British phonetician Henry Sweet. This system was to be used to represent the sounds of all the languages of the world and allowed phoneticians a system to communicate with each other.

1

If our spoken speech could accurately be represented by the English alphabet, then we would have no need for a phonetic alphabet. Let's take a brief look at how we spell and pronounce some common English words. Although we have only some 40 sounds in English, we have more than 200 ways of spelling them using our alphabet. For example, the sound of "sh" has up to 14 different spellings (faction, shoot, sugar, mission, ocean, champagne, etc.), the long "o" sound can be represented by over a dozen spellings (crow, so, doe, beau, etc.), and the long "a" sound in our alphabet is represented by 12 different spellings (lay, take, maid, freight, great, hey, etc.). Many consonants also are represented in several different ways. Consider the spelling of "t" in thank, tender, notion, the "h" in ache, hoist, hour, three, and enough, and the "c" in chair, bloc, and citrus. Although there has been a constant push from various groups to regularize our spelling, these movements have been met with resistance for centuries. You can see that mastery of the phonetic alphabet is an absolute necessity for anyone who needs an unambiguous, one-to-one representation of spoken speech. The phonetic alphabet meets this need.

Phonetic symbols are placed in slash marks or virgules such as /k/. Brackets [ ] are used to indicate a group of connected speech sounds.

Many consonant symbols of the IPA originate from the Roman alphabet: p, b, t, d, k, g, l, m, n, r, f, v, s, z, and w. Other symbols are from the Greek alphabet or have been created especially for the IPA. The "x" is not found in the IPA and is represented by /ks/, as "q" is represented by /kw/. Similarly, the "c" is represented by a /k/ in words with a "k" sound.

The Greek capital Theta /θ/ is used for the voiceless "th" as in "**th**igh." The /ð/ represents the voiced "th" as in "**th**is." An upside down "w" /ʍ/ or /hw/ is used for the voiceless "wh" as in "**wh**eat."

A lengthened sigmoid /ʃ/ represents the "sh" as in "**sh**ip." The /ʒ/ symbolizes the "zh" sound as in "bei**ge**." The IPA combines the symbols /t/ and /ʃ/ into /tʃ/ for the "ch" sound as in "**ch**ick." Similarly, the /d/ and /ʒ/ join for /dʒ/ as in "**J**ack." The symbol /ŋ/ represents the "ng" sound as in "ri**ng**." The /j/ may look familiar to you, but in the IPA it is used to represent the "y" sound as in "**y**oung." IPA symbols for English consonants are shown in Table 1–1.

The vowels of the IPA may be considered more challenging than the consonants as you must learn a new sound/symbol system for the majority of them. For instance, the "a, e, i, u" do not represent the traditional vowel sounds. In addition, the IPA uses /ɪ/ /ʊ/ /æ/ /ɛ/ /ɝ/ /ɚ/ /ʌ/ /ə/ /ɔ/. You will be relieved to learn that the "o" is represented by the familiar /o/ in the IPA, although some phoneticians use the /oʊ/ to represent "o." As you can see, the vowels of the IPA can be confusing. Similarly, the diphthongs present another sound difference. The diphthongs are written as a combination of two vowel sounds fused together, for example, the /aɪ/ in the word "island." Other diphthongs include /aʊ/ as in "**ou**t," /ɔɪ/ as in "**co**y," and /ju/ as in "**cu**te." IPA symbols for English vowels and dipthongs are shown in Table 1–2.

You are learning a new, exciting language—it will take time and study, but your efforts will be rewarded as you master transcription with the IPA!

Why Is It Important to Study Phonetics?

Phonetics, the study of speech sounds, is an extremely useful (and mandatory!) tool for the speech-language pathologist. The *Inter-*

Table 1–1. English Consonants and Their IPA Symbols

Primary Allographic or Orthographic Symbol	IPA Symbol	Key Words
p	/p/	pal, apart, tap
b	/b/	barn, cabin, rub
t	/t/	tea, water, aunt
d	/d/	dish, lady, sand
k	/k/	card, bacon, hook
g	/g/	game, sugar, bag
f	/f/	feed, afford, elf
v	/v/	van, envy, have
th	/θ/	thin, something, cloth
th	/ð/	this, weather, bathe
s	/s/	sat, lesson, horse
z	/z/	zone, puzzle, hose
sh	/ʃ/	ship, fashion, mash
zh	/ʒ/	treasure, beige
h	/h/	hit, behave
wh	/hw/	which, nowhere
ch	/tʃ/	chip, scratching, pitch
j	/dʒ/	jam, magic, page
w	/w/	wet, sandwich
y	/j/	yard, beyond
l	/l/	leaf, mellow, hill
r	/r/	rake, carrot, or
m	/m/	men, camel, time
n	/n/	net, dinner, pine
ng	/ŋ/	ringer, ring

national *Phonetic Alphabet* (IPA) is used to transcribe, or record using the IPA, the speech of a client. Transcribing the speech errors of a child or adult is an integral part of the assessment process.

Transcription can be *phonemic* or *phonetic*. Phonemic transcription is broad transcription. Broad transcription converts speech into phonemic symbols, written with virgules / /. Phonetic transcription is narrow transcription which records exactly how an utterance was produced. Narrow transcription utilizes diacritics (see Chapter 15), indicating a specific way a phoneme was produced. Words are written in brackets [ ].

Recording of the client's speech using the IPA enables another professional to identify how speech sounds have been produced.

Table 1–2. English Vowels and Their IPA Symbols

Primary Allographic or Orthographic Symbol	IPA Symbol	Key Words
ee	/i/	eat, keep, free
-i-	/ɪ/	in, mitt, city
-e-	/ɛ/	ebb, net
-a-	/æ/	at, bat, ham
a-e	/e/	age, face, say
-ur-	/ɝ/ (stressed)	earn, herd, fur
	/ɚ/ (unstressed)	herder, percent
-u-	/ʌ/ (stressed)	up, cup, done
	/ə/ (unstressed)	alive, relative, sofa
-oo-	/u/	boot, stew, soup
-oo-	/ʊ/	hood, could, cook
-aw-	/ɔ/	all, yawn, paw
-o-	/ɑ/	on, bomb
oa	/o/	oak, pole, toe
ou	/aʊ/	ouch, gown, how
i-e	/aɪ/	ice, shine, rye
oi	/ɔɪ/	oyster, loin, toy
u	/ju/	use, cue, mew

How Speech Sounds Can Be Studied

One of the ways in which speech sounds can be studied is as isolated, separate, and independent entities. Another way speech sounds can be studied is by comparing one sound with another sound. In this Workbook, we will discuss the system of speech sounds classified as Standard American English (SAE), the major dialect of English spoken in the United States of America. Refer to Chapter 16 for a definition of SAE.

A detailed study of speech sounds involves three reference points: (a) the organs that produce speech and their function in producing speech sounds *(physiological phonetics)*, (b) the physical properties of the individual speech sounds *(acoustic phonetics)*, and (c) the process by which the individual speech sounds are perceived and identified *(perceptual phonetics)*. Physiological phonetics is the focus of this Workbook as discussed in Chapter 2.

Regardless of the setting in which a speech-language pathologist is employed, a thorough knowledge of phonetics is essential. For instance, it is not uncommon for a speech-language pathologist employed in a school setting to use phonetics daily. Considering the importance of phonetics as a *functional* tool, it has always puzzled the authors that only one semester of undergraduate phonetics is required for majors in speech-language pathology in the United States. In the United Kingdom, four courses in phonetics are required!

STUDY QUESTIONS

1. Why is mastery of the International Phonetic Alphabet (IPA) important?

Phonetic transcript is narrow transcript which
records exactly how an utteran is pronovnce

2. From what language did many of the IPA symbols originate?

- English - Greek - Roman

3. What is the purpose of the IPA?

To transcribe the utterance of a word
Sound/sybol system used to represent the sounds of all language

4. Why are the IPA vowels considered more challenging than the consonants?

diphthong : must learn new sound/symbol system for
majorit of IPA word

5. Define Phonetics.

The study of speech and sound

6. Name and describe the three reference points in the study of speech sounds.

* Sound perception (Perceptual phonetics) ● Physical properties of speech sound (Acoustic phonetic)
● Organ that produce speech & function (Physiological phonetics)

7. Write the IPA phoneme which represents the following sounds:

a. "sh" _ʃ_

b. "th" _ð_ and _θ_

c. "ng" _ŋ_

d. "ee" _i_

e. schwa _tʃ_

f. "ash" _æ_

8. What is the difference between _phonemic_ and _phonetic_ transcription?

phonemic - no use of diacritic marks to speify how speech sound

2

Learning to Write
IPA Symbols
Syllables and Word Shapes

Learning Objectives

After reading this chapter, you will be able to:

1. Define a syllable and its components.

2. Explain the difference between a closed and open syllable.

3. Define Initial-Medial-Final consonant position.

4. State why it is essential to write IPA symbols correctly.

5. Write consonants, vowels, and diphthongs of IPA correctly.

Studying this chapter will familiarize you with the symbols of the IPA and how to write them correctly. The only way to become comfortable with writing the unfamiliar symbols is to practice, practice, practice! In addition, exercises are provided for you to learn the distinction between the spelling of a word (orthography) and how the word *sounds*.

An important part of learning phonetics is the ability to identify the position of a phoneme in a word. Terms used to describe

the position of a sound in a word vary. Words can be divided into syllables, with "V" indicating a vowel and "C" indicating a consonant. For example, the word "sold" is a one-syllable word with the CVCC classification. An example of a two-syllable word is "soda," which would be identified as CVCV.

Consonants have been viewed as appearing in one of three positions in a word: at the beginning of a word (*initial position*) or the first sound heard, the middle of a word (*medial position*), and at the end of a word *(final position)* or the last sound heard. Another classification system identifies a consonant that occurs *before* a vowel as a *prevocalic* consonant, one that occurs *between* two vowels as an *intervocalic* consonant, and a consonant that occurs *following* a vowel as a *postvocalic* consonant. Locate the /l/ phoneme in the words "look," "alone" and "cool":

Initial Position or Prevocalic: look

Medial Position or Intervocalic: alone

Final Position or Postvocalic: cool

The prevocalic and postvocalic classification system is useful in classifying position of consonant clusters. A *cluster*, also known as a *blend*, is two or more consonants within the same syllable. These can occur in prevocalic or postvocalic positions. Table 3–4 in the following chapter provides examples of consonant clusters.

Recently, consonant locations have been described in terms of their functions rather than their specific location in a word. Consonants can be viewed as performing only two functions, *releasing* vowels or *arresting* vowels. In the word "soap" the consonant /s/ releases the vowel /o/ while the consonant /p/ stops or arrests the vowel.

Bernthal and Bankson (1998) specify the *initial, medial, final* word position as the system used most often for sound-position descriptors. In this Workbook, an initial, medial and final identification exercise has been provided for each IPA phoneme. The words in these exercises were selected to increase your listening ability and to reinforce the difference between the way a word is spelled and how it is pronounced. You will find that the specific phoneme may not always occur in the word examples. These exercises can be heard on the audio CDs. Students who are learning English as a second language should find these exercises particularly useful.

Learning to Write IPA Symbols: Syllables and Word Shapes

One goal of this chapter is that you will learn to write the symbols of the IPA correctly and learn the sound/symbol association, which is the foundation of phonetics.

Directions for Study Card Use

The Phoneme Study Cards that accompany this book are an essential tool in the mastery of the sound/symbol association of the International Phonetic Alphabet.

Each card is numbered. Corresponding numbers are cited in the Transcription Exercises to help you identify the phoneme. You can also listen to the pronunciation of the Study Card on CD 2, Tracks 42–88.

Here are some suggestions for using these cards:

1 Learn the **sound** of the IPA phoneme shown on the front of the card. Remember that you can listen to the sounds pronounced on the audio CDs.

2 Memorize the phonetic description for each phoneme.

3 Become familiar with the word-position examples.

4 Create phonetically transcribed words by using the cards.

5 Challenge yourself to reduce the amount of time it takes to identify the sound of each phoneme.

6 Drill, drill, drill!

Following are examples of IPA phonemes. The phoneme is handwritten for you and you can practice writing the phoneme in the space provided.

The "Familiar" IPA Consonants

It is *essential* that you write the symbols of the IPA correctly. If you do not write the symbols correctly, another professional will not be able to read your transcription (Figure 2–1). This is critical because all your referrals: (1) to yourself during reassessment and treatment, (2) to your professional colleagues, and (3) to your supervisors must exactly reflect the same information.

"P/p" is written as   p

"B/b" is written as   b

"K/k" is written as   k

"G/g" is written as   g

"T/t" is written as   t

"D/d" is written as   d

"S/s" is written as   s

"Z/z" is written as   z

"W/w" is written as   w

"F/f" is written as   f

"V/v" is written as   v

"R/r" is written as   r

"J/j" is written as   j

"H/h" is written as   h

"L/l" is written as   l

"M/m" is written as   m

"N/n" is written as   n

Figure 2–1. Familiar IPA consonants.

The "Unfamiliar" IPA Consonants

These consonants may seem very strange, but you will become much more at ease with them as you continue your study of phonetics (Figure 2–2).

The Vowels of the IPA

The vowels of the IPA may seem confusing at first, but practice will help (Figure 2–3)! Remember: Do not be confused by spelling, but keep in mind the *sound* of the vowel.

How Do I Write the /æ/?

1 Write the schwa, starting at the top of the letter (Figure 2–4).

2 Without lifting your pencil from the paper, continue writing the letter "e."

"sh" as in "*sh*ip" is written as   ʃ

"zh" as in "bei*ge*" is written as   ʒ

"th" as in "*th*in" is written as   θ

"th" as in "*th*is" is written as   ð

"ng" as in "si*ng*" is written as   ŋ

"ch" as in "*ch*urch" is written as   tʃ

"j" as in "*j*am" is written as   dʒ

Figure 2–2. Unfamiliar IPA consonants.

The short "i" as in "zip" is written as   ɪ _____

The long "e" as in "keep" is written as   i _____

The short "e" as in "bet" is written as   ɛ _____

The short "a" as in "cat" is written as   æ _____

The long "a" as in "ape" is written as   e _____

The "ah" sound as in "sod" is written as   ɑ _____

The "uh" sound as in "cup" is written as   ʌ _____

The schwa as in "*a*bout" is written as   ə _____

The "oo" as in "soup" is written as   u _____

The "oo" as in "c*oo*k" is written as   ʊ _____

The "o" as in "boat" is written as   o _____

The "aw" as in "paw" is written as   ɔ _____

The "er" as in "h*er*d" is written as   ɜ _____

The "er" as in "herd*er*" is written as   ɚ _____

Figure 2–3. Vowels of the IPA.

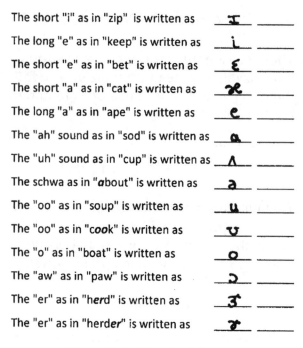

1. ə   ð   2. æ   æ

Figure 2–4. Writing the ash.

"ie" as in "p*ie*" is written as   aɪ _____

"ou" as in "c*ow*" is written as   aʊ _____

"oy" as in "b*oy*" is written as   ɔɪ _____

"u" as in "v*iew*" is written as   ju _____

Figure 2–5. Diphthongs of the IPA.

How to Write the Capped /a/ Used in Dipthongs

1 Write the curved line.

2 Add the half circle.

1: ⌐↓

2: ϛC

Completed: a   a

- Add the /ɪ/ and a diphthong to make the rising low front to high front off-glide diphthong: aɪ
- Add the /ʊ/ and a diphthong to make the rising low front to high back off-glide diphthong: aʊ

Figure 2–6. How to write the /a/.

The Diphthongs of the IPA

The diphthongs present their own unique challenge because two vowels are used. In addition, the diphthongs are written with a slur (‿) beneath them. See Figure 2–5. It is important to write the "a" of the diphthongs correctly. Figure 2–6 will help you.

Syllables

An important part of learning phonetics is the ability to identify the position of a phoneme in a word. Syllables comprise words. Hegde (2007) states that children and adults can identify syllables in words, but cannot define a syllable. A syllable can be formed by one *vowel*, *diphthong*, or *syllabic consonant* (see Chapter 5 regarding syllabic consonants). In addition, a *consonant* and vowel or diphthong can form a syllable. Vowels and diphthongs are produced by an unobstructed breathstream. Consonants are formed with an obstructed or partially obstructed vocal tract. A syllable includes the *onset* (a consonant that releases the *nucleus* of the syllable) and the *rhyme*. The rhyme consists of two parts, the nucleus (vowel) and the *coda* or consonant that may added at the end of the vowel. For example, for the word "sat" (consisting of one syllable), the onset is the consonant /s/, and the rhyme consists of the nucleus vowel /æ/, plus the coda or consonant /t/. It is convenient to call the consonant /s/ the *releaser* of the nucleus vowel and /t/ the *arrester* of the nucleus vowel. In addition, syllables can be closed (containing a coda) or open (no coda).

Here's a trivia question: What entertainment icon dropped a syllable from her name before she became famous? Answer: Barbara (Bar-ba-ra) Streisand eliminated a syllable to become Barbra (Bar-bra). (Mann, 2012).

Table 2–1 provides examples of different types of syllables.

Here are some words divided into syllables to study as examples:

1. phone   (1)
2. phoneme   (2) phon-eme
3. phonetics   (3) pho-net-ics
4. phonetician   (4) pho-ne-ti-cian
5. university   (5) un-i-vers-i-ty

Table 2–1. Syllables

		RHYME (Vowel and Coda)			
		Onset (Consonant Before Vowel)	**Nucleus** (Vowel)	**Coda** (Consonant After Vowel)	**Orthographic**
	1.	p	æ	n	pan (1)
	2.	s	i		sea (2)
	3.		ɪ	t	it (1)
	4.	spr	ɪ	ŋ	spring (1)
	5.	p	ɔ		paw (2)
	6.	θ	ɑ	t	thought (1)
	7.	skr	i	tʃ	screech (1)
	8.		a̯ɪ	l	I (2)
	9.	n	a̯ʊ		now (2)
	10.	t	ʌ	f	tough (1)

(1) = Closed syllables (contains coda).
(2) = Open syllable (contains no coda).

Exercise 2–A.

Now it's your turn. Divide these words into syllables. (Answers in Appendix B)

	Syllable Division	**# Syllables**
1. coda	co-da	2
2. nucleus	nu-cle-us	3
3. vowel	vow-el	2
4. syllable	syl-la-ble	3
5. rhyme	ryhme	1
6. initial	i-ni-tial	3
7. medial	me-di-al	3
8. final	fi-nal	2
9. blend	blend	1
10. cluster	clus-ter	2
11. arresting	ar-rest-ing	3
12. releasing	re-leas-ing	3
13. consonant	con-so-nant	3
14. orthography	or-thog-ra-phy	4
15. pound	pound	1
16. wiggle	wig-gle	2
17. intelligence	in-tel-li-gence	4
18. mathematical	mathe-mat-ical	5
19. centimeter	cen-ti-me-ter	4
20. chocolate	choc-o-late	3

Another system used to identify consonants and vowels in words is by using "C" for a consonant and "V" for a vowel. For example, the word "sold" is a one syllable word with a CVCC classification. An example of a two syllable word is 'soda," with a CVCV classification. Table 2–2 provides examples of word syllable shapes.

Table 2–2. Word Syllable Shapes

Cluster: Two adjacent consonants in the same syllable				
sing:	**C**	**V**	**C**	
	s	ɪ	ŋ	
singing:	**C**	**V**	**C**	**V**	**C**
	s	ɪ	ŋ	ɪ	ŋ
sting:	**C**	**C**	**V**	**C**	
	s	t	ɪ	ŋ	
string:	**C**	**C**	**C**	**V**	**C**
	s	t	r	ɪ	ŋ

C = Consonant; **V** = Vowel.

Exercise 2–B.

Provide the syllable shapes for these words. The first three have been completed for you. Check your answers in Appendix B.

What syllable shapes fit the following words?

1. ash   V C

2. crash   C C V C

3. splash   C C C V C

4. eastern   V V C C V C C

5. green   C C V V C

6. three   C C C V V

7. preach   C C V V C C

8. scream   C C C V V C

9. frame   C C V C V

10. phosphorus C C V C C C V C V C

Exercise 2–C.

Here's a challenge. Exercise 2–C lists dinosaur names. Put these in CV shapes. Answers in Appendix B.

What syllable shapes fit the following dinosaur names?

1. Brachyceratops   ccvcccvcvcvcc

2. Corythosaurus   cvccc cvcvvcvc

3. Dilophosaurus   cvcvccvcvvcvc

4. Microceratops   cv ccvcvcvcvcc

5. Pachyrhinosaurus   cvc cc ccvcvcvvcvc

6. Pentaceratops   cvccvcvcvcvcc

7. Triceratops   ccvcvcvcvcc

8. Brachiosaurus   ccvccvvcvvcvc

9. Epachthosaurus   vcvccccvcvvcvc

10. Heterodontosaurus   cvcvvcvccvcvcvc

Transcription Exercise 2–1.   **Track: (CD 1, Track 2)**

It is important that you develop the skill to determine the number of *sounds* contained in a word. Count how many sounds each word contains. Listen to CD 1, Track 2 to hear these words pronounced. The Examples section should be helpful to you.

Examples

noisy has 4 sounds: n ɔɪ z i

cough has 3 sounds: k ɑ f

together has 6 sounds: t u g ɛ ð ɚ

ship has 3 sounds: ʃ ɪ p

knife has 3 sounds: n aɪ f

giraffe has 4 sounds: dʒ ɚ æ f

baked has 4 sounds: b e k t

phantom has 6 sounds: f æ n t ə m

might has 3 sounds: m aɪ t

anniversary has 9 sounds: æ n ɪ v ɚ s ə r i

write has 3 sounds: r aɪ t

long has 3 sounds: l ɑ ŋ
Note: "ng" is transcribed: ŋ

whole has 3 sounds: h o l

"x" has 3 sounds: ɛ ks

measure has 4 sounds: m ɛ ʒ ɚ

gnat has 3 sounds: n æ t

Sounds		Transcription
2	1. gnaw	[n ɔ]
3	2. shape	[ʃ e p]
5	3. cousin	[k ʌ z ɪ n]
4	4. leisure	[l i ʒ ɚ]
3	5. tongue	[t ʌ ŋ]
2	6. who	[h ʊ]
4	7. rather	[r æ ð ɚ]
3	8. tough	[t ʌ f]
3	9. kneel	[n i l]
3	10. ax	[æ k s]
7	11. cinnamon	[s ɪ n ʌ m ɪ n]
3	12. wrap	[r æ p]
4	13. raked	[r e k t]
3	14. sight	[s aɪ t]
5	15. phoneme	[f o n i m]

Transcription Exercise 2–2.   **Track: (CD 1, Track 3)**

Phoneme Fill-In Exercise

Directions: Using the IPA, write the first *sound* in each of the following words:

1. push   p
2. real   r
3. act   æ
4. key   k
5. top   t
6. in   I
7. see   s
8. every   ɛ
9. very   v
10. urge   ɝ
11. easy   i
12. dog   d
13. able   e

Write the letters and see what they spell:

Transcription Exercise 2–3. **Track: (CD 1, Track 4)**

Phoneme Identification Exercise

This introductory exercise in phoneme identification is designed to fine-tune your listening abilities. Listen to each word and write the phoneme common to each group of words.

Remember—don't let spelling confuse you!

Consonants　　　　　　　　　　　　　　　　　　　　　　**Phoneme**

1. chorus	Quaker	mannequin	Zachary	physique	/_k_/
2. tango	kangaroo	Hong Kong	mingle	rectangle	/_ŋ_/
3. jumbo	effigy	geology	damage	fugitive	/_dʒ_/
4. phrase	raffle	tough	factory	Ralph	/_f_/
5. yesterday	papaya	Johann	bayou	savior	/_j_/
6. misery	hose	adviser	weighs	resume	/_z_/

Vowels

7. fruit	loop	tube	knew	zoos	/_u_/
8. eve	cease	free	quiche	beanie	/_i_/
9. coach	own	robe	beau	throw	/_o_/
10. birch	hermit	urge	myrtle	fur	/_ɝ_/
11. bathe	lay	vein	gate	eighty	/_e_/
12. ah	jaunt	spa	palm	shock	/_ɑ_/

YOUR FIRST EXERCISE—Transcribe Your Name!

Transcription Rules

Rule 1: Transcribe according to the way your name *sounds,* not how it is *spelled.*

Rule 2: No capital letters for your first, middle, or last name.

Rule 3: Put first, middle, and last names in one set of brackets: [   ].

Rule 4: No double phonetic symbols—remember, it is how your name sounds, not how many letters are used.

Helpful Hints

- Be sure to use the Study Cards to help you make the sound-symbol connection.
- Your phonetics instructor can review your transcription and make helpful suggestions.

JUST FOR FUN

Transcribe the names of family members, pets, favorite actors, and sports figures.

STUDY QUESTIONS

1. In word formations, what do "C" and "V" represent?

Consant

Vowel

2. List and define three consonant positions in words.

Initial: First sound heard   *final: Last sound heard at end of the word*

Medial: Sound in middle of a word

3. Define prevocalic, intervocalic, and postvocalic.

#1: Consonant preceding a vowel   *#3: Consonant after a vowel*

#2: Consonant occuring between two vowels

4. Define nucleus, onset, and coda.

#1: Vowel of syllable   *#3: Consonant after a vowel*

#2: Consant that realses the nucleus of a syllable

5. What comprises a syllable?

A vowel, diphthong or syllabic consonet

6. Give an example of a closed and open syllable.

Open: see

Closed: meet

7. Give an example of a CCCVC word.

sss Strap

8. Define orthography.

How a word is spelled

CHAPTER

3

Articulatory Aspects of Phonetics

Learning Objectives

After reading this chapter, you will be able to:

1. Name the four processes of PARR.

2. Describe vocal fold position for abduction and adduction.

3. Explain difference between place and manner of phoneme production.

4. State place and manner for all IPA consonants.

5. Define and give examples of syllable-initiating and syllable-terminating consonant clusters.

A review of basic anatomy and physiology is helpful for the beginning phonetics student as a basic understanding of speech production provides a necessary background for production of each phoneme. Keep in mind that this chapter provides a *brief* review.

The study of phonetics that describes the physiological properties of speech is called *physiological phonetics*. Various speech organs, such as the tongue, lips, teeth, and soft palate, can be positioned to create a wide variety of speech sounds simply by making small adjustments in the movements and locations of the speech organs within the oral cavity. These movements are performed automatically in the accomplished speaker and may become extremely complex in form.

The primary purpose of the structures used for speech is survival. For example, the lungs are the source of respiration, but they also provide a breathstream for speech. The tongue helps move the bolus of food to the posterior portion of the mouth so that the food can be swallowed, but it also produces speech sounds. The body parts used for speech production can be considered a

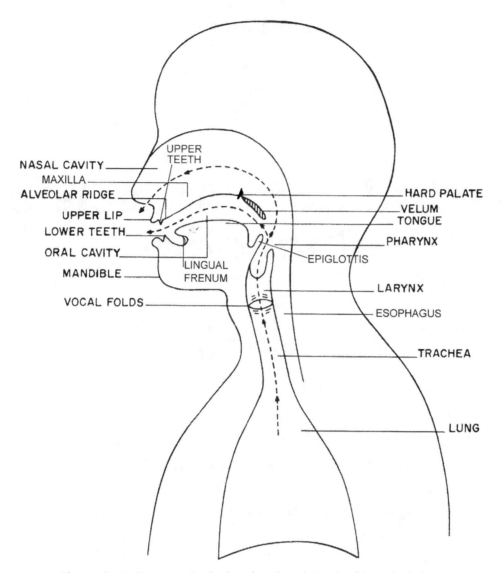

Figure 3–1. Structures in the head and neck involved in articulation.

speech-producing mechanism. Refer to Figure 3–1 and Figure 3–2 for an illustration of these body parts.

Larynx: The larynx is located in the throat, just above the trachea. It extends to the top of the esophagus, which is below the root of the tongue. Housed in the larynx are the *vocal folds.* The space between the vocal folds is the *glottis.* When the vocal folds **adduct,** or *close,* they vibrate to provide voicing for speech. When the folds **abduct,** or *open,* they do not vibrate and voicing is not produced.

Refer to Figure 3–3 for an illustration of the vocal folds.

Pharynx: A tubular, funnel-shaped structure located posterior to the root of the tongue and extending downward to the esophagus. The pharynx is divided into three parts: the nasopharynx, oropharynx, and the laryngopharynx (see Figure 3–2).

Nasopharynx: Section of the pharynx that lies directly posterior to the nasal cavity. Extends anteriorly from the nostrils to the posterior wall of the pharynx.

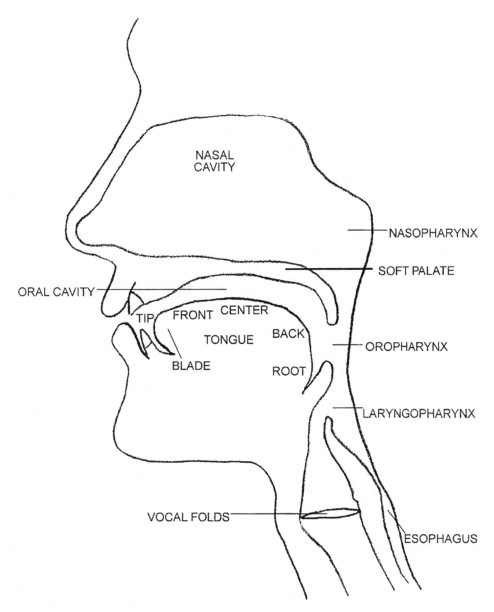

Figure 3–2. Resonating cavities and tongue.

Oropharynx: Section of the pharynx that is directly posterior to the oral cavity and extends from the level of the velum above to the level or the root of the tongue below. Can be easily viewed when the mouth is wide open and the tongue is pulled forward.

Laryngopharynx: The lower part of the pharynx that lies directly behind the laryngeal structures.

The pharynx contains two valves: the velopharyngeal valve and the epiglottal valve.

Velopharyngeal valve: Located at the juncture of the oropharynx and the nasopharynx. When this valve activates, it closes the nasopharynx and obstructs the laryngeal airstream from entering the nasopharynx and the nasal cavity.

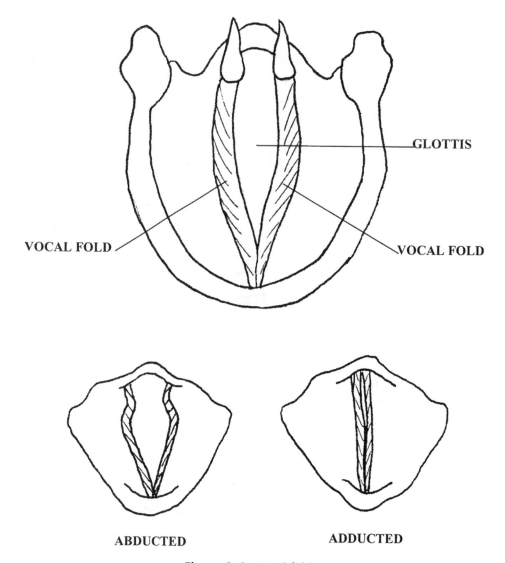

Figure 3–3. Vocal folds.

Epiglottal valve: Located just below the root of the tongue at the juncture of the oropharynx and the laryngopharynx. The epiglottis acts like a cover for the opening of the larynx during the passage of food from the oral cavity into the esophagus.

Oral cavity: The *oropharynx* opens anteriorly into the *oral cavity.* The oral cavity is bounded anteriorly by the lips and laterally by the cheeks. The tongue rests on the floor of the oral cavity. The hard palate and the velum form the roof of the oral cavity.

Lips: The upper and lower lips are made of muscles that have a great degree of mobility, facilitating the formation of various lip shapes for the production of vowels such as /ɑ,o,ʊ,æ/ and consonants, such as /p,b,m,w,hw,f,v/.

Teeth: The upper and lower teeth lie posterior to the lips. The upper and lower incisors, in particular, play an important role in the production of some consonants. The consonants involving both upper and lower incisors are /θ,ð/ and the consonants involving only the lower incisors are /f,v/.

Alveolar ridge: These ridges are located in the maxilla and mandible and contain the upper and lower teeth. The area directly behind the upper anterior teeth is commonly referenced for production of lingua-alveolar consonants. It serves as the point of contact or approximation for the tongue tip or front of the tongue in the production of numerous speech sounds such as the /t,d,l,s,z/.

Hard palate: The anterior two thirds of the roof of the mouth is arched and comprises the bony *hard palate*. The hard palate serves as the point of contact, or the point of approximation, for the front of the tongue in the production of speech sounds such as /ʃ,ʒ,j/.

Velum: The posterior one third of the palate. It is soft and muscular. It is also known as the soft palate. The velum serves as the point of contact for the back of the tongue in the production of speech sounds such as /k,g,ŋ/. The velum, aided somewhat by the posterior pharyngeal wall musculature, forms a valve known as the *velopharyngeal valve.*

This valve opens and closes the port between the nasopharynx and the oropharynx. When the valve is open, the speech sounds produced have a nasal resonance caused by the passage of a portion of the laryngeal airstream through the nasal cavity, as in the production of English consonants /m,n,ŋ/. However, the valve is usually closed during the production of speech sounds that do not require nasal resonance, as in the production of English vowels and non-nasal consonants.

Tongue: Derived from the Latin word *"lingua,"* the tongue is an exclusively muscular organ that rests on the floor of the oral cavity. It is an extremely mobile organ capable of making innumerable changes in positioning and muscle tension guided by the action of the intrinsic (originating inside the tongue) and extrinsic (originating outside the tongue muscles). All vowels are influenced by tongue position. The only consonants that do not have direct tongue involvement are: /m,p,b,f,v/.

Lingual frenum: Small, white cord of tissue. This tissue extends from the floor of the oral cavity to the midline of the under surface of the tongue blade. A frenum that is too short may restrict production of sounds which require tongue elevation.

Maxilla: The upper jaw which forms the majority of the palate.

Mandible: The lower jaw. Helps to move the lower teeth close to or away from the upper teeth. Its movement helps to reduce or enlarge the size of the oral cavity. The maximum downward movement of the mandible is seen during the production of the English vowel /æ/.

Lungs: The lungs are the organ of respiration and provide a breath stream for speech. Speech is produced when the breath stream is exhaled, or expelled, from the lungs.

Trachea: Rings comprised of cartilage and membranes leading from the larynx into the lungs; often referred to as the "windpipe."

Speech Processes

Speech is the end product of the four processes of Phonation, Articulation, Respiration, and Resonance (PARR).

Phonation is accomplished with the rhythmic and rapid opening and closing of the vocal folds, which open or close the glottis.

Articulation is how the breath stream is modified to form speech sounds.

Respiration provides the flow of air for speech, which is exhalation.

Resonation is the process of vibrating air in a resonating cavity. The resonating cavities were discussed earlier in this chapter.

Articulatory Aspects of Consonants

The production of consonants can be described by the *place* of articulation (*where* the phoneme is produced), the *manner* of articulation (*how* the breath stream is modified as it passes through the oral cavity), and *voicing* (if the vocal folds adduct for a voiced phoneme or abduct for an unvoiced phoneme). The majority of the consonants of the IPA are *cognates*, which means the phonemes are made in the same place and in the same manner, with the only difference being in voicing.

Each phoneme in the IPA is identified by place, manner, voicing, and distinctive features. Distinctive features are discussed later in this chapter. As you review each phoneme page, you will find the phoneme described by manner, place, voicing, and distinctive features.

Place of Articulation

Figure 3–4 illustrates the oral cavity shapes for the places of articulation.

Bilabial: Sounds produced at the lips are known as *labial* sounds. The English phonemes /p/, /b/, /m/, /w/, and /hw/ are classified as bilabials because both (or *bi-*) lips are used to produce them. The upper and lower lips serve as *articulators*, which are movable speech organs involved in the shaping of speech sounds. Only the lower lip is involved in production of /f/ and /v/.

Labiodental: The /f/ and /v/ phonemes are classified as *labio-* (meaning lip) *-dental* (meaning teeth) as the lip and teeth produce those phonemes.

Linguadental: *Lingua-* (meaning tongue) *-dental* (teeth) sounds are produced when the tip of the tongue is between the upper and lower teeth. These phonemes /θ/ and /ð/ are also referred to as interdentals, reflecting the tongue tip position between the upper and lower teeth.

Alveolar: The *alveolar* ridge (see Figure 3–1) is a very important point of tongue contact in many world languages, including English. Numerous sounds are produced when the tongue tip touches the alveolar ridge. The /t/, /d/, /n/, /s/, /z/, /l/, and /r/ are classified as lingua-alveolar phonemes.

Palatal: The consonants /ʃ/, /ʒ/, /tʃ/, /dʒ/, and /j/ are produced by the body of the tongue contacting, or approximating, the posterior portion of the hard palate.

Velar: The consonants /k/, /g/, and /ŋ/ are classified as lingua-velar sounds when the back portion of the tongue contacts the velum, or soft palate.

Glottal: The /h/ phoneme is classified as a glottal because it is produced when the vocal folds partially adduct to create friction or turbulence. The tongue does not assume any specific position in the oral cavity, and may be in position to produce the sound that follows the /h/.

Table 3–1 summarizes place of articulation. Table 3–2 summarizes place and manner.

Manner of Articulation

Manner of articulation describes *how* speech sounds are produced. The articulators are

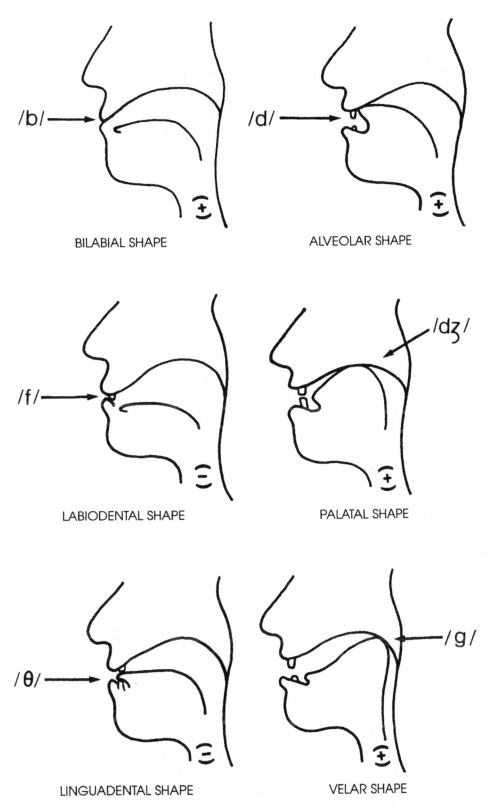

Figure 3–4. Diagram showing the six different alterations in the oral cavity shape controlled by lip and tongue contacts at the six different places along the horizontal line of the oral cavity. Plus sign (+) indicates presence of voicing; minus (–) sign indicates absence of voicing.

Table 3–1. Places of Articulation

CONSONANT	PLACE OF ARTICULATION	ARTICULATORS
/ p, b, m, w /	Bilabial	Lips
/ f, v /	Labiodental	Lower lip and upper teeth
/ θ, ð /	Linguadental	Tip of tongue and teeth
/ t, d, n, s, z, l, r /	Alveolar	Tip of tongue and alveolar ridge
/ ʃ, ʒ, tʃ, dʒ, j /	Palatal	Body of tongue and hard palate
/ k, g, ŋ /	Velar	Back of tongue and soft palate
/ h /	Glottal	Adduction/abduction of vocal folds

Table 3–2. Consonants Arranged by Place and Manner

Manner: →						
Place: ↓	Stop/Plosive	Fricative	Nasal	Affricate	Glides	Liquids
Bilabial	/p/(−), /b/(+)		/m/(+)		/w/(+)	
Lingua-Alveolar	/t/(−), /d/(+)	/s/(−), /z/(+)	/n/(+)			/l/(+)
Linguavelar	/k/(−), /g/(+)		/ŋ/(+)			
Labiodental		/f/(−), /v/(+)				
Interdental		/θ/(−), /ð/(+)				
Glottal		/h/(−)				
Labial-Velar		/hw/(−)				
Linguapalatal		/ʃ/(−), /ʒ/(+)			/j/(+)	
Alveo-Palatal				/tʃ/(−), /dʒ/(+)		/r/(+)

(+) Indicates a voiced phoneme.
(−) Indicates an unvoiced phoneme.

positioned and must react in a specific way to produce the phoneme. Ways in which consonants are produced are described by the terms in Figure 3–5. Looking at this figure, you will note that a consonant can belong to more than one category.

See Exercises 3–A through 3–E for practice identifying manner of articulation.

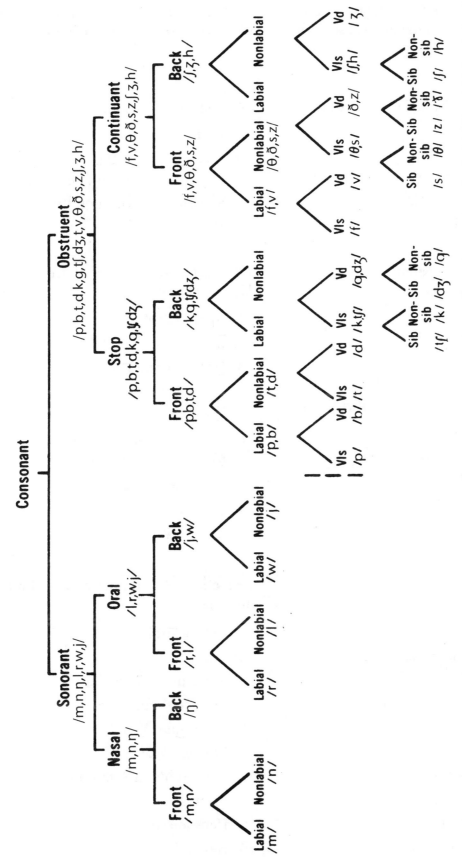

Figure 3–5. Division of consonants, on binary principles, into sonorant/obstruent, nasal/oral, stop/continuant, front/back, labial/nonlabial, voiceless/voiced (Vls/Vd), and sibilant/nonsibilant (Sib/Non-Sib) groups. (Reproduced with permission from *Phonetics: Principles and Practices* [3rd ed.], by S. Singh and K. Singh, 2006, p. 63. Copyright 2006 Plural Publishing, Inc.)

Exercises 3–A through 3–E give you an opportunity to identify *manner of articulation*. Circle the consonant(s) in each song title. All of these songs were recorded and/or written by the Beatles. Answers in Appendix B.

Exercise 3–A. Manner of articulation: *Stop-Consonants*

1. Blackbird
2. Day Tripper
3. Get Back
4. Paperback Writer
5. Ticket to Ride
6. A Hard Day's Night
7. I Got to Find My Baby
8. I'll Be Back
9. Come and Get It
10. Let It Be

Exercise 3–B. Manner of articulation: *Nasals*

1. If I Needed Someone
2. Lady Madonna
3. Lend Me Your Comb
4. Maggie Mae
5. Penny Lane
6. Sun King
7. Taxman
8. Honeymoon Song
9. Tip of My Tongue
10. Mailman, Bring Me No More Blues

Exercise 3–C. Manner of articulation: *Fricatives*

1. Another Girl
2. Strawberry Fields Forever
3. Dizzy Miss Lizzy
4. Good Day Sunshine
5. Here Comes the Sun

6. I Saw Her Standing There
7. If I Fell
8. I've Just Seen a Face
9. Lucy in the Sky with Diamonds
10. She Came in Through the Bathroom Window

Exercise 3–D. Manner of articulation: *Liquids and Glides*

1. Eleanor Rigby
2. Lovely Rita
3. Yellow Submarine
4. Words of Love
5. Young Blood
6. Ballad of John and Yoko
7. Watching Rainbows
8. Winston's Walk
9. Yesterday
10. Run for Your Life

Exercise 3–E. Manner of articulation: *Affricates*

1. Act Naturally
2. Julia
3. Magical Mystery Tour
4. Mother Nature's Son
5. Norwegian Wood
6. Blue Jay Way
7. Baby You're a Rich Man
8. Chains
9. Her Majesty
10. Hey Jude

Obstruents: Obstruents are produced with an *obstruc*tion in the vocal tract, which can be a complete or incomplete obstruction.

Sonorants: A sonorant is the opposite of an obstruent because the sound passes through a relatively open channel and is not blocked.

Stops: These phonemes are produced with a total blockage of the airstream. In these consonants, the airstream must be released after it is blocked. This class of consonants is also referred to as plosives.

Continuants: Unlike the stops, continuants are produced in a *continu*ing manner, with relatively less obstruction. Contrast production of the /t/ as in "tuh, tuh, tuh," with the continuous flow of air when producing the /s/ as in "s-s-s-s-s."

Fricatives: These phonemes are obstruents because they are produced with a partial blockage of the airstream, resulting in turbulence or *fric*tion.

Affricates: The only affricates in the IPA, /tʃ/ and /dʒ/, begin with production of a stop-consonant and end with production of a fricative.

Orals: This category refers to resonating cavities (see Figure 3–2). The consonants in this group are produced in the resonating cavity of the vocal tract excluding the nasal cavity and nasopharynx.

Nasals: The /m/, /n/, and /ŋ/ are the only consonants requiring nasal resonance. The resonating cavity is the entire vocal tract, including the nasal cavity and the nasopharynx. Nasal resonance is accomplished by the lowering of the velum to permit airflow into the nasal cavity.

Liquids and glides: The consonants /ɾ/, /l/, /w/, and /j/ are considered liquids and glides because of their extreme flexibility in assuming the role of either a consonant or a vowel. The /l/ is also called a lateral because it is the only phoneme with airflow around the *sides* of the tongue.

Voiced and voiceless: This category focuses on the vibration of the vocal folds. For a voiced phoneme, the vocal folds are *ad*ducted and vibrate. For voiceless sounds, the vocal folds are *ab*ducted and no voicing is produced.

Articulatory Aspects of Vowels

Vowel classification differs greatly from the system used to classify consonants. Vowels are classified by tongue position (refer to Figure 9–1). All vowels require voicing produced by the vibrating vocal folds. Refer to Chapter 9 for more information about vowels.

Distinctive Features

Distinctive features are those attributes of a phoneme that are required to differentiate one phoneme from another in a language. For example, the phonemes /k/ and /g/ in English are differentiated by the feature of voicing, which in turn is an attribute in differentiating phonemes in the English language. Figure 3–6 displays distinctive feature contrast for English consonants. The features are:

Voicing/voiceless: The vocal folds *ad*duct for a voiced phoneme and *ab*duct for a voiceless phoneme.

Front/back: The consonant is produced in the front of the vocal tract (lips, alveolar ridge) or in the back of the vocal tract (hard or soft palate).

Labial/nonlabial: One or both lips are used in producing the consonant or the lips are not used to form the sound.

Sonorant/nonsonorant: The relatively open vocal tract is used to produce a sonorant consonant; nonsonorant refers to an obstructed vocal tract.

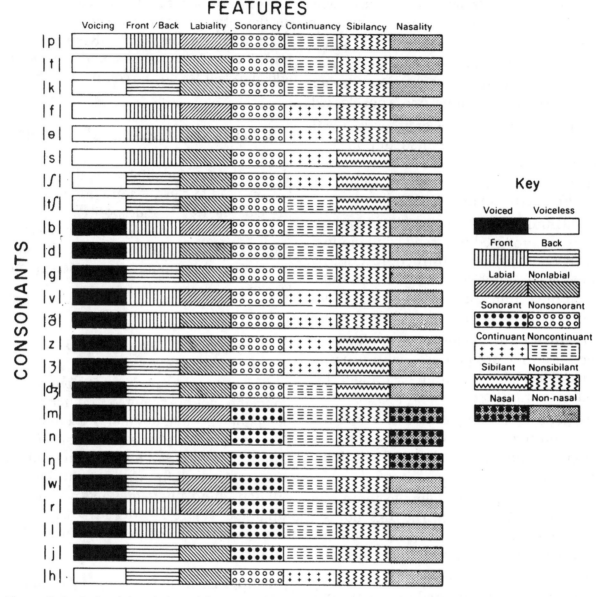

Figure 3–6. A visual description of distinctive feature contrast among English consonants. (Reprinted with permission from *Phonetics: Principles and Practices* [3rd ed.], by S. Singh and K. Singh, 2006, p. 168. Copyright 2006 Plural Publishing, Inc.)

Continuant/noncontinuant: Continuant phonemes are made without a constriction so that the airflow is not blocked. A noncontinuant sound is constricted.

Sibilant/nonsibilant: Consonants with this distinctive feature have a "hissing" sound such as the /s/ or /ʃ/.

Nasal/non-nasal: Nasal consonants require nasal resonance through lowering of the velopharyngeal port to allow the airflow into the nasal cavity.

Ages of Consonant Development

Table 3–3 presents data summarized from several studies indicating ages of consonant development. You will note variation in age of acquisition of the various consonants.

Table 3–3. Developmental Norms for Phonemes

Phonemes	Wellman et al. (1931)	Poole (1934)	Templin (1957)	Sander (1972)	Prather et al. (1975)	Arlt et al. (1976)	Fudala & Reynolds (1986)	Smit et al. (1990)
m	3	3½	3	≤ 2	2	3	2 ½	≤ 3½
n	3	4½	3	≤ 2	2	3	2	≤ 3½
h	3	3½	3	≤ 2	2	3	1½	≤ 3
p	4	3½	3	≤ 2	2	3	2	3 to 3½
f	3	5½	3	3	2 to 4	3	2 ½	3½ to 4
w	3	3½	3	≤ 2	2 to 8	3	1½	≤ 3
b	3	3½	4	≤ 2	2 to 8	3	2	≤ 3
ŋ	—	4½	3	2	2	3	—	≥ 9
j	4	4½	3½	3½	3	3	3	3½ to 4
k	4	4½	4	2	2 to 4	3	2½	≤ 4
g	4	4½	4	2	2 to 4	3	2½	3 to 4
l	4	6½	6	3	2 to 4	4	5	5 to 6
d	5	4½	4	2	2 to 4	3	2½	≤ 3½
t	5	4½	6	2	2 to 8	3	3	≤ 3½
s	5	7½	4½	3	3	4	11	9
r	5	7½	4	3	3 to 4	5	5½	8
tʃ	5	—	4½	4	3 to 8	4	5½	5½ to 7
v	5	6½	6	4	4+	3½	5½	4½ to 5½
z	5	7½	7	4	4+	4	11	≥ 9
ʒ	6	6½	7	6	4	4	—	—
θ	—	7½	6	5	4+	5	5½	6 to 7
dʒ	—	—	7	4	4+	4	5	6 to 7
ʃ	—	6½	4	4	3 to 8	4½	5½	6 to 7
ð	—	6½	7	5	4	5	5½	4½ to 7

Consonant Clusters

A *consonant cluster*, also referred to as a *consonant blend*, is a combination of two or more adjacent consonants in the same syllable. The words "tree" [tri] and "street" [strit] have double and triple consonant clusters, respectively, in the initial position of the word. Clusters can also occur in the medial position (underlined) as in "restrain" [ristren] or in the final position as in "fast" [fæst].

A consonant cluster is simply a way of combining the consonant phonemes in a language. Only certain consonants can be used to form clusters. While initial consonant clusters /st/, /sk/, /sp/, and /sw/ occur in English, clusters such as /sb/, /sd/, /sg/, /sr/, and /sv/ are not found in the initial position of a word in English. Table 3–4 provides numerous examples of clusters in Standard American English in the initial (syllable-initiating) and final (syllable-terminating) positions.

Table 3–4. Examples of Consonant Clusters in American English

Consonant Cluster	Word Examples	Consonant Cluster	Word Examples
Syllable Initiating (Initial)		**Syllable Terminating (Final)**	
bl-	bleak, blame, black	-ft	left, lift, soft
fl-	flake, flag, flee	-gz	wigs, rags, bugs
gl-	glad, glow, gleam	-ks	lacks, walks, likes
kl-	clean, clap, close	-kt	pact, fact, act
pl-	plan, pleat, plow		
sl-	sleep, slide, slender	-lb	bulb
		-ld	mold, bald, sold
br-	brain, bring, brag	-lf	elf, calf, shelf
dr-	dress, drink, drip	-lk	walk, elk, milk
fr-	frame, frost, fright	-lp	help, gulp, pulp
gr-	grin, grape, grip	-lt	salt, fault, malt
kr-	cry, creep, crop	-lz	sells, malls, wheels
pr-	price, practical, pro		
tr-	trim, treat, trick	-mp	stamp, jump, bump
shr-	shred, shrub, shrine	-mpt	stomped, jumped, bumped
thr-	through, threat, throw	-mps	lamps, ramps, jumps
		-mz	arms, stems, aims
sk-	scoop, schedule, skim		
skr-	scream, screech, scrap	-nd	hand, bend, wind
skw-	squeal, squash, squander	-ndz	hands, bends, grounds
		-nt	ant, rent, print
sm-	smile, smear, smug	-nts	prints, joints, ants
		-nz	plans, runs, burns
sn-	sneak, snow, sniff		
		-ŋk	junk, sank, bank
sp-	speak, spot, sparkle	-ŋz	kings, wings, sings
spl-	splash, splendor, split		
spr-	sprout, spring, spruce	-pt	roped, seeped, shopped
st-	stew, stop, steel	-rd	guard, sword, hard
str-	strike, street, stripe	-rf	scarf
		-rk	fork, shark, mark
kw-	queen, quantity, quiver	-rm	charm, form, dorm
		-rn	learn, fern, barn
sw-	sweet, swipe, swat	-rst	first, worst, burst
tw-	twin, twenty, tweezer	-rt	cart, sort, art
fj-	few, future, fume	-rv	carve, starve, nerve
kj-	cute, cube, accuse	-st	nest, past, test
mj-	music, amuse, stimulate	-ts	mats, bets, sits

STUDY QUESTIONS

1. What is the primary purpose of the structures used for speech?

   Survival functions

2. Define PARR.

   Phonation Articulation Respiration Resonation

3. How do place and manner of articulation differ?

   Place: Speech Sound is produced (location)

   manner: How the speech sound is produced

4. How do nasals gain resonance?

   Nasal Cavity

5. What is the difference between adducted and abducted vocal folds?

   #1: Vocal folds Close & Vibrate

   #2: Vocal folds open & don't vibrate

6. Fill in the anatomic structure associated with production of:
   a. Bilabials   lip
   b. Glottals   Glottis
   c. Linguadentals   tounge, upper & lower teeth
   d. Alveolars   Alveolar ridge
   e. Palatals   hard palate
   f. Velars   Velum or Soft palate

7. What is a cluster or blend?

   2 or 3 Consonant in the Same

   Syllable

8. What is the difference between an obstruent ① and a sonorant ②?

#1: Obstruction of vocal tract

#2: open channel not blocked

4

Stop-Consonants

Learning Objectives

After reading this chapter, you will be able to:

1. Explain the two phases of production of a stop-consonant.

2. Define a glottal stop and voiced /t/ and the difference in place and manner of production.

3. Identify cognates of /p/t/k/.

4. Transcribe words using stop consonants.

Stop-consonants, also known as plosives, require a stopping of the breathstream by a closure within the oral cavity. Production of a stop-consonant is a *manner* of articulation. Manner of articulation was discussed in Chapter 3. There are two phases involved in production of a stop-consonant: the air must be stopped and then it must be released. Stopping of the air is mandatory, as air must be held in the oral cavity. The plosive phase of the stop releases the impounded air. Stopping of the airstream can occur by lip closure, as in producing /b/, tongue elevation, as in production of /t/, or by adduction of the vocal folds for a glottal stop.

Release of the air, also known as aspiration, can occur in two ways. The air can be released as a "puff" of air, similar to that of an ex*plosion*, when released into a vowel as in the word "pay" [pʰe] or released without the explosion of air as in the phrase "at work." The symbol [ʰ] identifies aspiration of the impounded air and the [ˋ] denotes unreleased air.

Edwards (2003) discusses "The Strange Case of the American English /t/" and lists ten allophonic variations. An allophonic variation is a difference in the way a phoneme can be produced. The /t/ does differ from other English consonants because of its many variations. For example, the /t/ may be voiced, substituted with a glottal stop, or intruded in a word. You have transcription exercises for some of these variations in this chapter.

/p/

Transcription Exercise 4–1   **Track: (CD 1, Track 5)**

		I	M	F
1.	phone			
2.	split		✗	
3.	hiccough		✗	✗
4.	gopher			
5.	shopping		✗	
6.	president	✗		
7.	peppermint	✗	✗	
8.	pneumatic			
9.	append		✗	
10.	pamphlet	✗		

Transcription Exercise 4–2
Consonant: /p/

 Track: (CD 1, Track 6)
Refer to Study Card: 3

Phonetic Symbol	Target Word	Transcription
/p/	1. pine	paɪn
	2. deep	dip
	3. oppose	ə'poz
	4. cape	kep
	5. paper	pepɚ
	6. sip	sɪp
	7. place	ples
	8. help	hɛlp
	9. pack	pæk

/p/

Distinctive Features	Tongue Position
Bilabial stop consonant Voiceless, front, labial, nonsonorant, noncontinuant, nonsibilant, non-nasal 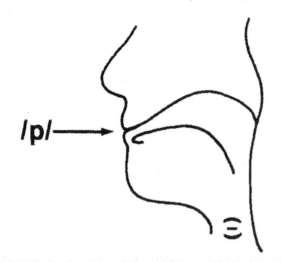	Not relevant for production of this phoneme. May be in position for following consonant or vowel. Lips are closed. Breath is held and compressed in oral cavity. Breath stream may or may not be released with aspiration; dependent upon surrounding consonants and syllable position.

Voicing/Velopharyngeal Port	Spelling Variations
Voiceless—vocal folds *ab*duct. VP port is closed.	Appears as /p/ in words Appears in clusters with /l/r/s/spl/spr/ pp in medial position (*apply/o*ppose) is transcribed with a single /p/ This phoneme may be intruded in the following words if an unvoiced phoneme follows a nasal: warmth [wɔrmpθ] comfort [kʌmpfɚt] dreamt [drɛmpt]

Word Position	Clinical Information
Initial, medial, and final positions in SAE	Cognate of /b/

/b/

Transcription Exercise 4–3   **Track: (CD 1, Track 7)**

		I	M	F
1.	humble		X	
2.	ribbon		X	
3.	belabor	X	X	
4.	public		X	
5.	Burbank	X	X	
6.	thumb			
7.	probe			X
8.	halibut		X	
9.	broke	X		
10.	tombstone			

Transcription Exercise 4–4
Consonant: /b/

 Track: (CD 1, Track 8)
Refer to Study Card: 4

Phonetic Symbol	Target Word	Transcription
/b/	1. bad	bæd
	2. tub	tʌb
	3. baby	bebi
	4. bright	braɪt
	5. rabbit	ræbɪt
	6. nobody	nobɑdi
	7. bomb	bɑm
	8. cob	kɔb
	9. curb	kɝb

/b/

Distinctive Features	Tongue Position
Bilabial stop consonant Voiced, front, labial, nonsonorant, noncontinuant, nonsibilant, non-nasal /b/ →	Irrelevant; tongue may be in position for following consonant or vowel. Lips are closed. Breath is held and compressed in oral cavity. Breath stream may or may not be released with aspiration; dependent upon surrounding consonants and syllable position.
Voicing/Velopharyngeal Port	**Spelling Variations**
Voiced—Vocal folds *ad*duct. VP port is closed.	bb in medial position (ho*bb*y, ru*bb*er) is transcribed with a single /b/ pb occurs rarely as /b/ in cu*pb*oard silent /b/ in bom*b*
Word Positions	**Clinical Information**
Initial, medial, and final positions in SAE	Cognate of /p/

Crossword Puzzle for /p/ and /b/

Answers in Appendix B

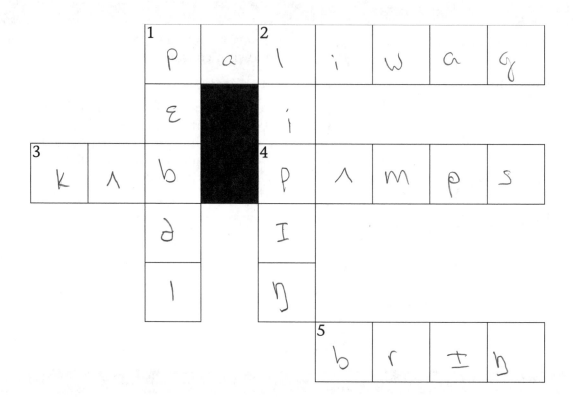

Directions: Transcribe the following words:

Across:

1. pollywog
3. cub
4. pumps
5. bring

Down:

1. pebble
2. leaping

BABYTIME

Word Search #1 Answers in Appendix B

```
s  ʃ  r  d  aɪ p  ɚ  z  d  ɔ  l  t  z  r
d  ʒ  ɚ  k  ʃ  ə  b  p  æ  n  d  ə  ð  ʌ
b  ɑ  t  ə  l  o  r  r  i  æ  k  n  ʊ  d
s  tʃ i  w  b  l  u  p  m  ɪ  p  z  n  kʍ
h  p  ɛ  t  e  v  i  b  b  e  u  l  m  p
f  ɑ  ʒ  ŋ  b  ɛ  ʌ  ɔ  k  r  ɪ  p  t  s
k  p  t  θ  i  p  z  z  t  dʒ i  b  v  n
l  ɑ  s  l  z  ð  w  k  m  æ  ʒ  n  æ  p
b  ɛ  f  o  ɪ  ɛ  r  ʃ  ɪ  k  o  u  r  æ
h  b  æ  s  ɪ  n  ɛ  t  r  g  l  ʊ  f  s
n  ɪ  z  ɛ  g  ɔ  ɪ  ʌ  i  d  r  s  n  ɪ
s  b  e  b  ɪ  b  n  z  b  ʌ  n  i  g  f
p  ɪ  ŋ  k  w  dʒ ð  b  e  ʌ  ɛ  ɪ  ʒ  aɪ
j  f  e  ɪ  w  ə  p  r  w  ɝ  g  v  z  j
l  b  l  æ  ŋ  k  ɛ  t  p  t  d  i  ɔ  ɚ
r  g  h  p  ks f  m  ɚ  b  g  ɑ  r  ə  g
```

Directions: Find and circle the words listed below which contain the /p/ or /b/ phonemes.

papa	pacifier	bunny	bassinet
panda	bib	diapers	blanket
pink	bottle	blue	nap
baby			

/t/

Transcription Exercise 4–5   Track: (CD 1, Track 9)

		I	M	F
1.	caught			✗
2.	whistle			
3.	tuition	✗		
4.	thyme	✗	✗	
5.	tentative	✗	✗	
6.	tortilla	✗	✗	
7.	watched			✗
8.	chalet			
9.	territory	✗	✗	
10.	motion			

Transcription Exercise 4–6
Consonant: /t/

 Track: (CD 1, Track 10)
Refer to Study Card: 5

Phonetic Symbol	Target Word	Transcription
/t/	1. tube	tʌb
	2. cut	kʌt
	3. into	Intʊ
	4. until	ʌntIl
	5. twin	twIn
	6. coat	kot
	7. rotate	rotet
	8. time	tɑɪm
	9. nest	nɛst

/t/

Distinctive Features	Tongue Position
Lingua-alveolar stop-consonant Voiceless, front, nonlabial, nonsonorant, noncontinuant, nonsibilant, non-nasal 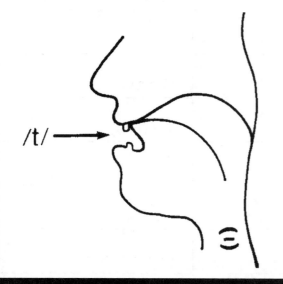	Tip of tongue contacts alveolar ridge with sides against upper molars. Breath is held in oral cavity; may be released with or without aspiration.
Voicing/Velopharyngeal Port	**Spelling Variations**
Voiceless—vocal folds *ab*duct. VP port is closed.	Usually occurs as /t/. tt transcribed as a single /t/ in medial position as in li*tt*le. -ed following unvoiced consonants as in wish*ed*, cough*ed*, tap*ed* is transcribed with a /t/, except following the /t/ as in ska*ted* or wai*ted*. th as in *Th*omas, *Th*eresa transcribed as /t/. n( )s results in an intruded /t/ sound, not included in spelling, between /n/ and /s/ as in chance [tʃæn^{t}s] or tense [tɛn^{t}s]. t is silent in sof*t*en, cas*t*le, whis*t*le.
Word Position	**Clinical Information**
Initial, medial, and final positions in SAE	Commonly replaced with the voiced /t/ or glottal stop Cognate of /d/ tr- in *tr*anquil or *tr*actor can be produced as the /tʃ/.

The Glottal Stop

Transcription Exercise 4–7   **Track: (CD 1, Track 11)**

Remember these things about the glottal stop:

1 It is an allophonic variation of the /t/ and /k/.

2 Do not confuse the glottal stop with a question mark. It is written as: ʔ

3 When followed by an "n" in the spelling of the word, a syllabic /ŋ/ is used.

The glottal stop is produced by the vocal folds when they *ad*duct to hold air in the glottis (space between the vocal folds) and *ab*duct to release the air. This exercise will give you an opportunity to hear the difference between production of the /t/ and the glottal stop.

Word	/t/ transcription	Glottal stop transcription
1. Doolittle	dulɪtəl	dulɪʔɪ
2. mitten	mɪtən	mɪʔn
3. fountain	faʊntən	faʊnʔn
4. patent	pætənt	pæʔnt
5. Hilton	hɪltən	hɪlʔn
6. button	bʌtən	bʌʔn
7. Latin	lætən	læʔn
8. cotton	kɔtən	kɔʔn
9. bitten	bɪtən	bɪʔn
10. molten	moltən	molʔn

The Voiced /t/

Transcription Exercise 4–8   🔾 **Track: (CD 1, Track 12)**

Like the glottal stop, the voiced /t/ is an allophonic variation of the /t/. It is an alternative pronunciation. The voiced /t/ can result when voiced phonemes precede and follow the /t/. In the examples that follow (with the exception of #3, "battle"), the /t/ is *intervocalic* (between two vowels), and the voiced sounds that surround the /t/ cause it to be voiced.

Voicing of the /t/ is dependent on syllable stress (see Chapter 14). If the second syllable containing the /t/ is not stressed, this allows for voicing of the /t/. Example: "total" could be transcribed as ['totǝl]. If the word is produced with stress on the second syllable containing the /t/, then the word is transcribed as [to'tǝl]. Pronounce these words: *detain*, *enter*, and *control*. These are examples of words with second syllable stress and the /t/ would not be voiced.

Accurate transcription is required to clarify what word the speaker has produced. For example, did the speaker say "bidder" [bɪdɚ] or "bitter" [bɪtɚ]? Narrow transcription of the /t/ is required to clarify which word was said for accurate transcription.

Transcribe the following words. Words in the first column are dictated with the /t/. The second column words are dictated with the voiced /t/. Remember that the voiced /t/ sounds like the /d/. Here is a rule for using a voiced /t/: *If a word is spelled with a "t," but you hear a "d," use the "v" (for voicing) /t̬/.*

Word	/t/ transcription	Voiced /t/ transcription
1. better	bɛˈtɚ	ˈbɛt̬ɚ
2. hotter	hɔtɚ	hɔt̬ɚ
3. battle	bæˈtǝl	bæt̬el
4. matter	mæˈtɚ	mæt̬ɚ
5. atom	æˈtǝm	æt̬ǝm
6. butter	bʌˈtɚ	ˈbʌt̬ɚ
7. cater	keˈtɚ	ket̬ɚ
8. quota	kwoˈtǝ	kwot̬ǝ
9. cheated	tʃitɪd	tʃit̬ɪd
10. duty	duˈti	ˈdut̬i

Some phoneticians use the alveolar flap (or tap) /ɾ/ to transcribe the voiced /t/. The term describes the tongue tip and blade briefly contacting, or flapping, against the upper alveolar ridge. Unlike production of the /t/, there is no build-up of air pressure. Shriberg and Kent (2012) describe the flap as a "modified stop." Edwards (2003) states the intervocalic /t/ can be transcribed as /t̬/ or /ɾ/. It is very difficult to *hear* the difference between a voiced /t̬/ or flap when words are produced. Ladefoged (2006) provides a detailed discussion of the alveolar flap. Test your listening skills: Listen to Elvis Presley sing "In the Ghetto." Do you hear Elvis sing the word as [ˈɡɛt̬o] or [ɡɛˈto]?

/d/

Transcription Exercise 4–9   **Track: (CD 1, Track 13)**

		I	M	F
1.	hedge			
2.	handkerchief			
3.	mapped			
4.	deadened	✗	✗	✗
5.	decade	✗		✗
6.	pointed			✗
7.	adding		✗	
8.	medial		✗	
9.	dread	✗		✗
10.	demand	✗		✗

Transcription Exercise 4–10
Consonant: /d/

 Track: (CD 1, Track 14)
Refer to Study Card: 6

Phonetic Symbol	Target Word	Transcription
/d/	1. dough	do
	2. condition	ˈkʌndɪʃən
	3. used	juzd
	4. dish	dɪʃ
	5. meadow	mɛdo
	6. sand	sænd
	7. dwell	dwɛl
	8. wonder	wʌndɚ
	9. changed	tʃendʒd

/d/

Distinctive Features	Tongue Position
Lingua–alveolar stop-consonant Voiced front, nonlabial, nonsonorant, noncontinuant, nonsibilant, non-nasal /d/ ⟶	Same as for the cognate /t/ As a voiced phoneme, less breath pressure is required than for voiceless /t/.

Voicing/Velopharyngeal Port	Spelling Variations
Voiced—vocal folds *ad*duct. VP port is closed.	d is primary. dd is transcribed with a /d/ as in a*dd* or sa*dd*er. -ed has sound of /d/ following vowels as in mow*ed* and pray*ed* and voiced consonants as in sav*ed* or open*ed*. ld occurs with silent /l/ in cou*ld*, shou*ld*.

Word Position	Clinical Information
Initial, medial, and final positions in SAE	Cognate of /t/ dr- in *dr*ive or *dr*ink can be produced as the /dʒ/.

Crossword Puzzle for /t/ and /d/

Answer in Appendix B

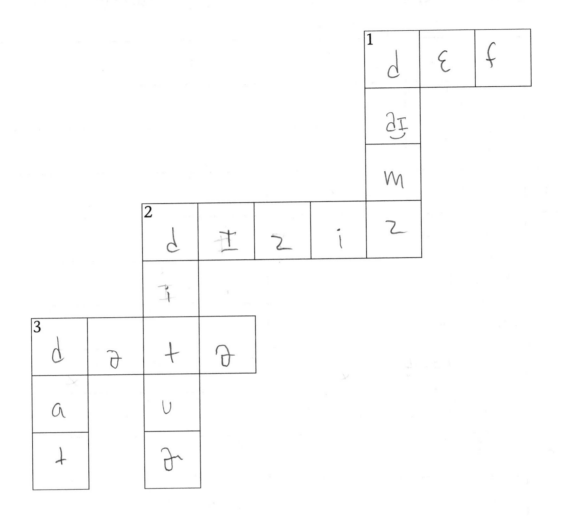

Directions: Transcribe the following words:

Across:

1. deaf
2. disease
3. data

Down:

1. dimes
2. detour
3. dot

/k/

Transcription Exercise 4–11   **Track: (CD 1, Track 15)**

		I	M	F
1.	centimeter		X	
2.	pique	X	X	
3.	quartet	X	X	
4.	text		X	
5.	bronchitis	X	X	X
6.	impeccable		X	X
7.	critic	X		X
8.	backache		X	X
9.	knight			
10.	Tocqueville		X	

Transcription Exercise 4–12
Consonant: /k/

 Track: (CD 1, Track 16)
Refer to Study Card: 1

Phonetic Symbol	Target Word	Transcription
/k/	1. back	bæk
	2. count	kaʊnt
	3. tick	tɪk
	4. basket	bæskɛt
	5. cake	kek
	6. cream	krim
	7. stocking	stakɪŋ
	8. across	əkras
	9. marquee	marki

/k/

Distinctive Features	Tongue Position
Lingua-velar stop consonant Voiceless, back, nonlabial, nonsonorant, noncontinuant, nonsibilant, non-nasal 	Back of tongue elevates to touch velum. Air pressure builds up behind tongue/velum seal. Lips are apart and neutral. Air pressure is released when tongue moves from velum.

Voicing/Velopharyngeal Port	Spelling Variations
Voiceless—vocal folds *abduct*. VP port is closed.	Numerous variations cc as in "occur" transcribed with a single /k/. ch as in *ache*, *ch*orus ck always has /k/ sound as in du*ck*, ti*ck* que as in techni*que* kh as in *kh*aki ng ( ) th results in an intruded /k/, not included in the spelling of the word, as in length. [lɛŋkθ] Cluster examples: kl, kr, sk, skw, skr

Word Position	Clinical Information
Initial, medial, and final positions in SAE	/t/ is often substituted for /k/ in young children. Cognate of /g/

/g/

Transcription Exercise 4–13   **Track: (CD 1, Track 17)**

		I	M	F
1.	gentle			
2.	garbage	✗		
3.	gnat			
4.	eggnog		✗	✗
5.	exist		✗	
6.	gouge	✗		
7.	laugh			
8.	Gertrude	✗		
9.	linger		✗	
10.	digit			

Transcription Exercise 4–14
Consonant: /g/

 Track: (CD 1, Track 18)
Refer to Study Card: 2

Phonetic Symbol	Target Word	Transcription
/g/	1. gone	gɑn
	2. wiggle	wɪgəl
	3. hungry	hʌngril
	4. beg	bɛg
	5. dog	dɔg
	6. green	grin
	7. vague	veg
	8. glove	glʌv
	9. griddle	grɪdəl

/g/

Distinctive Features	Tongue Position
Lingua-velar stop-consonant Voiced back, nonlabial, nonsonorant, noncontinuant, nonsibilant, non-nasal 	Same as for /k/ Produced with less breath pressure and muscular tension than /k/.
Voicing/Velopharyngeal Port	**Spelling Variations**
Voiced—vocal folds *ad*duct. VP port is closed.	gg transcribed with single /g/ sound. Exception: su*gg*est [sʌgdʒɛst] *gue* as in vo*gue* *gu* as in *gu*est, *gu*ard *gh* as in *gh*ost (e)x as in *exist* has the /gz/ sound [ɛgzɪst]
Word Positions	**Clinical Information**
Initial, medial, and final positions in SAE	Common articulatory substitution: d/g Cognate of /k/

Crossword Puzzle for /k/ and /g/

Answers in Appendix B

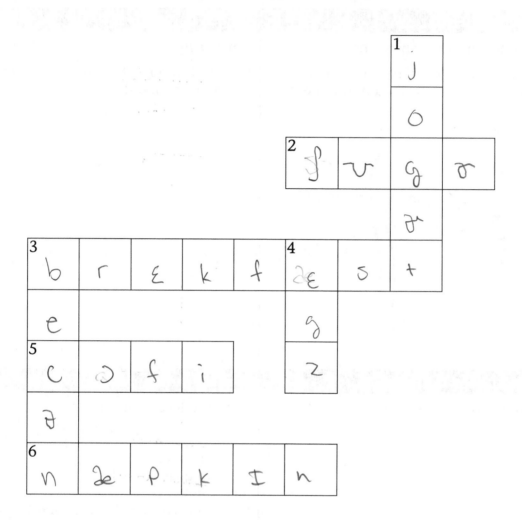

Directions: Transcribe the following words:

Across:

2. sugar
3. breakfast
5. coffee
6. napkin

Down:

1. yogurt
3. bacon
4. eggs

SPICE UP YOUR LIFE

Word Search #2   Answers in Appendix B

g   u   o   t   aɪ   m   b   k   ʌ   v   l   ɛ   k   t

k   ɔ   v   i   r   n   ʌ   t   m   ɛ   g   n   g   d

e   ʌ   d   ð   ɝ   ɝ   w   z   s   f   j   ɔ   t   ʃ

p   k   ɛ   k   i   k   ju   m   ɪ   n   h   ʒ   ɝ   o

ɚ   w   s   ɚ   ʌ   æ   ə   ɔ   h   l   e   h   m   ɛ

z   i   o   l   t   k   f   u   d   o   ɛ   m   ɚ   ɚ

e   k   ɛ   r   o   w   e   r   ɪ   t   ð   ɪ   ɪ   ʌ

h   s   r   æ   r   k   d   k   l   p   p   o   k   θ

k   f   t   k   ɛ   ɛ   v   m   t   r   t   l   p   n

r   k   m   d   g   r   k   ɔ   r   i   æ   n   d   ɚ

g   ɝ   æ   v   ə   t   r   o   ŋ   h   ɪ   t   b   m

b   i   ð   r   n   θ   p   æ   p   r   i   k   ə   g

o   ɪ   ɛ   k   o   g   t   n   ð   e   ʒ   æ   v   r

w   n   k   l   o   v   z   h   e   v   d   ɛ   g   j

f   tʃ   z   i   u   n   t   ɛ   r   ə   g   ɑ   n   ə

k   ɑ   r   d   ə   m   ə   m   ɛ   n   æ   t   tʃ   t

Directions: Find and circle the words listed below which contain the /t/d/k/ or /g/ phonemes.

caraway	turmeric	cumin	dill
cardamom	capers	oregano	coriander
curry	paprika	nutmeg	tarragon
thyme	cloves		

Stop-Consonant

Transcription Exercise 4–15
/ p / b / t / d / k / g /

Track: (CD 1, Track 19)
Phoneme Study Cards: 1–6

1. perpetrate   P3PItret
2. bucket   bʌkɪt
3. claypot   klepat
4. dropped   drapt
5. Pope   Pop
6. dot-to-dot   dat-tu-dat
7. cupcake   kʌpkek
8. babied   bebid
9. deadbolt   dɛdbolt
10. coat   kot
11. pagoda   pʌgodə
12. birdbeak   b3dbik
13. fixed   fɪkst
14. laptop   læptap
15. gabby   gæbi
16. dogtag   dɔgtæg
17. backup   bækʌp
18. toga   togə
19. pocketbook   pakItbʊk
20. kept   kɛpt

STUDY QUESTIONS

1. Name two phases of stop consonant production.

   Air stop in oral ; air is released

2. How is a glottal stop produced?

   Vocal folds adduct to hold air in glottis ;
   Vocal folds abduct to open & release air

3. How do consonant cognates differ?

   Only voicing differs

4. How is the alveolar flap/tap produced?

   tounge tip & blade briefly Contact
   or flaps, against upper Alveolar ridge

5. What are some allophonic variations of the /t/?

   Glottal stop voiced /t/ & alvedor flap

6. List the cognates for these stop consonants:

   a. /k/ _/g/_
   b. /t/ _/d/_
   c. /p/ _/b/_

7. List three things to remember about production of a glottal stop (refer to Transcription Exercise 4–7).

   All ophonic variation of /t/ & /k/
   - Not written as a question mark

   When glottal stop is followed by /n/, a syllabic /n/ is used

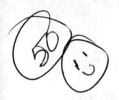

5

Consonants: Nasals and Syllabics

Learning Objectives

After reading this chapter, you will be able to:

1. Identify place of production of the nasal consonants.

2. State position of velopharyngeal port when a nasal is produced.

3. Define a syllabic consonant and give examples.

4. Explain the term "homorganic" and relationship to syllabic consonants.

5. List homorganic consonants for all nasals.

6. Transcribe words using nasal consonants.

Nasal Consonants

The nasal consonants are /m/n/ŋ/. They are the only consonants produced with nasal resonance. The velum is lowered, opening the velopharyngeal port to allow the breath-stream to enter the nasal cavity. Each nasal consonant differs in place of production. The /m/ is a bilabial and is produced with bilabial lip closure. Tongue position is not relevant for the /m/. The /n/ is produced with lingua-alveolar contact. The /ŋ/ is formed by the back portion of the tongue contacting the velum. All of the nasals are voiced.

/m/

Transcription Exercise 5–1   **Track: (CD 1, Track 20)**

		I	M	F
1.	mermaid	X	X	
2.	dime			X
3.	palm			X
4.	mum	X		X
5.	chasm		X	X
6.	minimum	X	X	X
7.	membrane	X	X	
8.	hammer		X	X
9.	squirm		X	X
10.	empire		X	

Transcription Exercise 5–2
Consonant: /m/

 Track: (CD 1, Track 21)
Refer to Study Card: 19

Phonetic Symbol	Target Word	Transcription
/m/	1. might	maɪt
	2. lamp	læmp
	3. meat	mit
	4. team	tim
	5. camera	kæmɚ
	6. malt	malt
	7. random	rændam
	8. harm	harm
	9. smell	smɛl

/m/

Distinctive Features	Tongue Position
Bilabial Nasal Voiced, front, labial, sonorant, noncontinuant, nonsibilant, nasal /m/→ — open velopharyngeal port	Tongue is flat in the oral cavity or is in place for the following phoneme. Lips are closed.

Voicing/Velopharyngeal Port	Spelling Variations
Voiced—vocal folds *ad*ducted. VP port is open—airflow through nasal cavity.	mm as in su*mm*er is transcribed with a single /m/. gm with silent /g/ as in diaphra*gm* mb with silent /b/ as in nu*mb* mn with silent /n/ as in hy*mn*

Word Positions	Clinical Information
Initial, medial, and final positions in SAE	Lips are brought together as for production of the bilabials /p/ and /b/. Homorganic (made in the same place) with /p/ and /b/.

/n/

Transcription Exercise 5–3   **Track: (CD 1, Track 22)**

		I	M	F
1.	knapsack	X		
2.	kennel		X	
3.	nonsense	X	X	
4.	zone			X
5.	gnash	X		
6.	pneumatic	X		
7.	noon	X		X
8.	gnome	X		
9.	beginner		X	
10.	seventeen			X

Transcription Exercise 5–4
Consonant: /n/

 Track: (CD 1, Track 23)
Refer to Study Card: 20

Phonetic Symbol	Target Word	Transcription
/n/	1. tennis	tɛnɪs
	2. cabin	kæbɪn
	3. noisy	nɔɪzi
	4. canary	kʌnɛri
	5. nautical	natɪkɒl
	6. violin	vaɪolɪn
	7. handy	hændi
	8. panel	pænal
	9. nylon	naɪlan

/n/

Distinctive Features	Tongue Position
Lingua-alveolar nasal consonant	Tip of tongue touches the alveolar ridge.
Voiced, front, nonlabial, sonorant, noncontinuant, nonsibilant, nasal	Front of tongue touches the upper alveolar ridge.
	Sides of tongue touch upper molars.
/n/→ **open velopharyngeal port**	Back of tongue is down.
	Teeth and lips are open.

Voicing/Velopharyngeal Port	Spelling Variations
Voiced—vocal folds *ad*ducted.	nn as in i*nn* transcribed with a single /n/
VP port is open—airflow through nasal cavity.	mn silent /m/ as in *mn*emonic
	pn silent /p/ as in *pn*eumonia
	kn silent /k/ as in *kn*ee
	gn silent /g/ as in si*gn*

Word Positions	Clinical Information
Initial, medial, and final positions in SAE	Homorganic (made in the same place) with /t/ and /d/.

TAKE TIME TO SMELL THE FLOWERS

Word Search #3   Answers in Appendix B

m	e	m	æ	g	n	o	l	j	ə	n
d	o	ə	p	k	dʒ	ɝ	i	e	ɪ z	ɛ
ɛ	f	o	r	dʒ	u	ʌ	p	ɛ	u ŋ	r
l	r	ð	ɪ	n	n	s	i	ɪ	o p	v
f	s	m	m	ʌ	m	t	t	u	o æ	θ
ɪ	p	ʃ	r	j	v	ks	u	ʊ	ɝ n	g
n	b	t	o	d	f	k	n	b	ɚ z	o
i	t	ɪ	z	e	p	ɑ	i	i	ə i	k
ə	d	s	o	m	ɛ	r	ə	g	o l	d
m	k	r	p	i	o	n	i	o	ʌ s	h
ə	g	ʊ	z	tʃ	w	e	ʒ	n	k s	ʒ
dʒ	æ	z	m	i	n	ʃ	z	i	g z	z
j	w	ɔ	ɪ	æ	n	ə	e	ə	s r	v
ʌ	z	ɪ	n	i	ə	n	w	o	z w	f

Directions: Find and circle the words listed below which contain the /m/ or /n/ phonemes.

mum	petunia	primrose
carnation	jasmine	zinnia
delphinium	magnolia	pansy
peony	begonia	marigold

/ŋ/

Transcription. Exercise 5–5   **Track: (CD 1, Track 24)**

		I	M	F
1.	monkey		✕	
2.	singing		✕	✕
3.	kingdom		✕	
4.	arrange			
5.	elongate		✕	
6.	wrong			✕
7.	jingle		✕	
8.	length		✕	
9.	fangs		✕	
10.	sponge			

Transcription Exercise 5–6
Consonant: /ŋ/

 Track: (CD 1, Track 25)
Refer to Study Card: 21

Reminder: Use /ɪ/ before "ing" words. See page 80

Phonetic Symbol	Target Word	Transcription
/ŋ/	1. bongo	bɔŋgo
	2. strongly	strɑŋli
	3. Hong Kong	haŋkan
	4. wing	wɪŋ
	5. tongue	tʌŋ
	6. shingle	ʃɪŋgəl
	7. dining	dɑɪnɪŋ
	8. fang	fɛŋ
	9. savings	sevɪŋz

/ŋ/

Distinctive Features	Tongue Position
Lingua-velar nasal consonant Voiced, back, nonlabial, sonorant, noncontinuant, nonsibilant, nasal 	Back of tongue is raised to contact velum. Sides of back of tongue contact back molars. Teeth and lips are open. Voice is directed through open VP port to nasal cavity.

Voicing/Velopharyngeal Port	Spelling Variations
Voiced—vocal folds *ad*ducted. VP port is open—airflow through nasal cavity.	Occurs as ng in words n (k) appears in mi*nk* [mɪŋk] or si*nk*. In the same syllable and often in adjoining syllables as in i*nc*ome [ɪŋkʌm]. ng as in si*ng*le [sɪŋəl] ngue as in to*ngue* [tʌŋ]

Word Positions	Clinical Information
Medial and final positions in SAE	Homorganic (made in the same place) with /k/ and /g/. Also called the "hooked n."

Why Use The /ɪ/ Before /ŋ/?

The high front vowel /ɪ/ is used to transcribe "ing" as in "making" [mekɪŋ] or "thing" [θɪŋ].

You may have the temptation to use the [i] before /ŋ/, but resist! Compare the difference between the sound of /i/ in "meat" [mit] or "three" [θri] to the /i/ in [iŋ] and you will hear that the vowel does not sound the same.

Another important consideration is the *phonetic environment* of the high front vowel when it is adjacent to a nasal sound. Phonetic environment is defined as the phonemes which surround a specific speech sound. The /ŋ/ is a nasal consonant which requires nasal resonance through opening of the velopharyngeal port. Since the "i" gains nasal resonance, it can also cause it to sound more like /ɪ/ rather than /i/.

Remember that this rule only applies to "i-ng" orthographically and not to any other vowels before "ng" as in "sang" [sæŋ] or "strong" [strɑŋ].

NASALS

Word Search #4   Answers in Appendix B

ʃ	d	l	ɔ	p	n	b	ʌ	dʒ	ʃ	ɪ	r	ʒ
æ	ŋ	k	ɚ	r	k	z	æ	ɝ	j	ɝ	ɛ	o
d	s	d	ʒ	t	θ	tʃ	ɪ	b	ɔ	b	k	ə
ɪ	ɑ	n	ɝ	ɔ	ʌ	r	m	r	h	ɝ	t	k
k	j	æ	ŋ	k	ɪ	ŋ	b	ɪ	ə	s	æ	b
d	t	k	d	l	ŋ	t	s	ŋ	o	l	ŋ	ɪ
ɪ	m	m	ʃ	ə	s	i	ɪ	k	ə	b	g	e
s	l	ɪ	ŋ	g	ɚ	m	tʃ	ə	i	z	ə	w
ŋ	k	ə	w	n	z	w	ʃ	e	tʃ	d	l	i
ʃ	l	ɪ	n	i	k	m	ʌ	ŋ	k	n	ð	æ
l	ɛ	h	ð	l	o	d	r	l	ɛ	s	t	t
ʃ	ŋ	l	o	ɪ	l	æ	e	e	o	d	ɛ	l
æ	k	m	tʃ	ŋ	g	b	s	w	ɪ	ŋ	z	i
p	θ	r	z	k	n	θ	ɪ	i	u	tʃ	d	z
h	ɪ	s	s	ʒ	s	r	ŋ	m	n	r	k	ɪ

Directions: Find and circle the words listed below which contain the /ŋ/.

linger	monk
length	racing
swings	rectangle
link	anchor
drink	yanking

Crossword Puzzle for /m/, /n/, and /ŋ/

Answers in Appendix B

1 n	aɪ	n		2 s
æ				t
p				i
3 k	ɪ	ŋ	d	ə	m
ɪ				
4 n	ʊ	m	o	n	j	ə

Directions: Transcribe the following words:

Across:
1. nine
3. kingdom
4. pneumonia

Down:
1. napkin
2. steam

Syllabics

In its simplest form, a syllabic is a consonant with a vowel-like quality. A syllabic consonant acts like a vowel. For example, the word "hidden" can be pronounced in two ways: (a) [hɪdən] or (b) [hɪdn̩]. In the first example, the tongue *leaves* the alveolar ridge after producing /d/ to produce the mid-central schwa vowel, and then returns to the alveolar ridge to produce /n/. In the second example, the tongue *remains* on the alveolar ridge after production of /d/ to produce the following syllabic /n̩/.

To change a consonant to a syllabic, a diacritic is used. A small vertical line (̩) is placed under the consonant. Remember that the diacritic (̩) *replaces* a vowel. No vowel will precede a syllabic consonant or appear in the same syllable where a syllabic occurs.

Use of syllabics is variable, depending on the speaker. Syllabics occur more frequently in conversational speech as they facilitate rapid rate of speech.

Syllabics serve as the center (nucleus) of a syllable. The /m̩/n̩/ŋ̍/l̩/ can function as a syllabic. Consonant syllabics function in unstressed syllables in words of two or more syllables. All vowels are syllabics.

Use of syllabics occurs in conversational speech and in producing the words in isolation, as in the example with "hidden." The /m̩/, /n̩/, and /ŋ̍/ syllabics share a homorganic (made in the same place of articulation) relationship with the previous phoneme. For example, the syllabic /m̩/ will follow /b/ and /p/ because they are made in the bilabial place of production. The syllabic /n̩/ can follow the lingua alveolar productions of /t/d/s/z/. The syllabic /ŋ̍/ can follow the lingua-velar /k/ and /g/. The syllabic /l̩/ can follow any consonant (Edwards, 2003). Examples of these syllabics:

	Word	Transcription
Syllabic /m/	open	[opm̩]
Syllabic /n/	reason	[rizn̩]
Syllabic /ŋ/	broken	[brokŋ̍]
Syllabic /l/	medal	[mɛdl̩]

Transcription Exercise 5–8 provides an opportunity to listen to syllabic consonants used in formal and casual speech.

Transcription Exercise 5–7
Nasal Consonants / m / n / ŋ /

 Track: (CD 1, Track 26)
Phoneme Study Cards: 19–21

1. nasal   nezəl

2. monumental manjumentəl

3. among   əmʌŋ

4. remnant   rɛmnɪnt

5. nominate   namInet

6. feminine   fɛmInIn

7. lemonade   lɛmoned

8. morning   mornɪŋ

9. chimney   tʃImni

10. meeting   mitIŋ

11. containing kʌntenIŋ

12. mingling   mIŋglIn

13. membrane   mɛmbren

14. money   mʌnI

15. nanny   næni

16. meringue   mʒen

17. mountain   maʊntIn

18. numerical numerIkəl

19. cinnamon   sInamʌn

20. moonbeam   munbim

Transcription Exercise 5–8   **Track: (CD 1, Track 27)**

This exercise will give you practice in identifying syllabics as used in formal and casual speech. The word will first be pronounced as it would in formal speech and then in casual speech. Listen carefully as some of these differences can be subtle. You may think that you've never said a word in that way, especially using syllabic /ŋ/ and /m̩/, but this is good practice. Words are transcribed for you in Appendix B.

	Formal Speech	Casual Speech
1. cabin	kæbɪn	kæbm̩
2. medal	mɛdəl	mɛdl̩
3. redden	rɛdɪn	rɛdn̩
4. ribbon	rɪbɪn	rɪbm̩
5. blacken	blækɪn	blækn̩
6. panel	pænəl	pænl̩
7. milking	mɪlkɪŋ	mɪlkŋ̩
8. garden	gardɪn	gardn̩
9. broken	brokɪn	brokŋ̩
10. open	opɪn	opm̩

STUDY QUESTIONS

1. What are the nasal consonants?

_____

_____

2. How does place of production for each of the nasal consonants differ?

_____

_____

3. Define homorganic.

_____

_____

4. What is a syllabic consonant?

_____

_____

5. Define the difference between formal and casual speech.

_____

_____

6. List the homorganic phoneme relationships for /n/m/ and /ŋ/.

_____

_____

7. What diacritic is used to indicate a syllabic? Give an example using a syllabic consonant.

_____

_____

CHAPTER

6

Consonants: Fricatives /s/z/f/v/ʃ/ʒ/θ/ð/h/hw/

Learning Objectives

After reading this chapter, you will be able to:

1. Explain the difference between production of stop consonants and fricatives.

2. State tongue and lip positions for interdentals and labiodentals.

3. List spelling variations for /f/.

4. Describe two tongue positions for /s/ and /z/.

5. Transcribe words using fricative consonants.

As discussed in Chapter 3, fricatives are produced when the breath stream passes through a narrow constriction in the vocal tract. Unlike the stop consonants that are produced with a complete obstruction of the breathstream, fricatives are produced with a *partial* blockage of the airstream.

Each fricative has a voiced cognate, with the exception of /h/ and /hw/. These phonemes are classified as fricatives but are not considered cognates as both phonemes are unvoiced when produced in isolation. Unlike the oral cavity, which is the source of friction for the majority of the fricatives, the glottis serves as the source of friction for the /h/ and /hw/.

/f/

Transcription Exercise 6–1   Track: (CD 1, Track 28)

		I	M	F
1.	phosphorus	✗	✗	
2.	pamphlet		✗	
3.	giraffe			✗
4.	photo	✗		
5.	fifteen	✗	✗	
6.	Joseph			✗
7.	spherical		✗	
8.	monograph			✗
9.	fluffy	✗	✗	
10.	phonograph	✗		✗

Transcription Exercise 6–2
Consonant: /f/

 Track: (CD 1, Track 29)
Refer to Study Card: 9

Phonetic Symbol	Target Word	Transcription
/f/	1. fun	fʌn
	2. before	bi for
	3. fifteen	fɪftin
	4. frost	frɑst
	5. coffee	kɔfi
	6. leaf	lif
	7. laugh	læt
	8. float	flot
	9. if	ɪf

/f/

Distinctive Features	Tongue Position
Labio-dental fricative Unvoiced, front, labial, nonsonorant, continuant, nonsibilant, non-nasal /f/ ⟶	Inner border of lower lip is raised to contact upper incisors. Breathstream is continuously emitted between upper teeth and lower lip, creating friction. Tongue position is irrelevant; may be in position for following phoneme.

Voicing/Velopharyngeal Port	Spelling Variations
Voiceless—vocal folds *ab*duct. VP port is closed.	ff is transcribed as single /f/ as in coffee. ph phone, prophet gh rough, laugh

Word Positions	Clinical Information
Initial, medial, and final positions in SAE	Common articulatory substitutions: p/f, b/f Cognate of /v/

/v/

Transcription Exercise 6–3   **Track: (CD 1, Track 30)**

		I	M	F
1.	vindictive	✓		✓
2.	wife			
3.	chevron		✓	
4.	weaver			✓
5.	of			✓
6.	lifesaving		✓	
7.	never		✓	
8.	wives		✓	
9.	verify	✓		
10.	stove			✓

Transcription Exercise 6–4
Consonant: /v/

 Track: (CD 1, Track 31)
Refer to Study Card: 10

Phonetic Symbol	Target Word	Transcription
/v/	1. vine	vaɪn
	2. velvet	vɛlvɪt
	3. over	ovɚ
	4. very	vɛri
	5. invite	ɪnvaɪt
	6. live	lɪv
	7. value	vælju
	8. weaver	wivɚ
	9. move	muv

/v/

Distinctive Features	Tongue Position
Labio-dental fricative Voiced front, labial, nonsonorant, continuant, nonsibilant, non-nasal /v/⟶	See /f/ for description of production.

Voicing/Velopharyngeal Port	Spelling Variations
Voiced—vocal folds *ad*duct. VP port is closed.	ph Ste*ph*en lv silent /l/ as in *calves, salves*

Word Positions	Clinical Information
Initial, medial, and final positions in SAE	Substituted with /b/ or omitted Cognate of /f/

Crossword Puzzle for /f/ and /v/

See Answers in Appendix B

1		2		3
k	æ	f	i	n
æ	■	ɛ		o
4 v	e	s		t
ɪ		t		ɪ
t		ɪ		f
i		v		aɪ
		ə		
5 f	l	ɪ	p	

Directions: Transcribe the following words:

Across:
1. caffeine
4. vase
5. flip

Down:
1. cavity
2. festival
3. notify

MONDAY NIGHT FOOTBALL

Word Search #5   Answers in Appendix B

v	ɪ	k	t	ɔ	r	i	h	e	d	ɪ	n
m	h	ɛ	g	d	e	t	r	r	b	s	h
ɑ	r	r	ɪ	t	ɚ	m	ɛ	i	n	k	ɛ
r	ɛ	ə	v	ɪ	n	s	k	s	ɑ	k	p
s	f	ʊ	t	b	ɔ	l	i	i	l	ɪ	d
u	ɚ	n	d	h	ɑ	r	v	v	i	k	ə
n	i	ə	s	e	f	t	i	ɚ	t	ɔ	h
b	l	u	d	w	ɪ	v	i	g	u	f	æ
f	ʊ	l	b	æ	k	l	ɑ	m	p	r	f
r	w	f	ɑ	d	s	w	r	θ	ɛ	e	b
ʊ	u	i	dʒ	d	ə	ʃ	s	ɛ	r	n	æ
k	d	l	u	æ	m	æ	ɪ	r	i	i	k
s	b	d	l	i	t	m	t	i	dʒ	ɛ	r
ɔ	f	ɛ	n	s	ɑ	d	i	f	ɛ	n	s

Directions: Find and circle the words listed below which contain the /f/ or /v/ phonemes.

referee	kickoff	fullback
football	varsity	field
victory	receiver	defense
safety	halfback	offense

/s/

Transcription Exercise 6–5   Track: (CD1, Track 32)

		I	M	F
1.	city	✗		
2.	shaves		✗	
3.	deceptive		✗	✗
4.	blintz			✗
5.	usual		✗	
6.	axes		✗	
7.	bracelet		✗	
8.	island			
9.	pseudo	✗		
10.	Bronx			✗

Transcription Exercise 6–6
Consonant: /s/

 Track: (CD 1, Track 33)
Refer to Study Card: 7

Phonetic Symbol	Target Word	Transcription
/s/	1. else	ɛls
	2. asleep	ə slip
	3. superior	supirijɚ
	4. basin	besɪn
	5. Easter	istɚ
	6. cedar	sidɚ
	7. asks	æsks
	8. sandal	sændʒl
	9. blast	blæst

/s/

Distinctive Features	Tongue Position
Lingua-alveolar fricative Voiceless, front, nonlabial, nonsonorant, continuant, sibilant, non-nasal 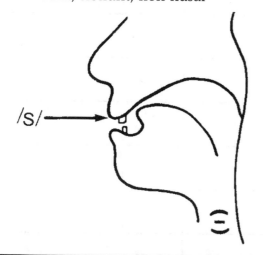	Tongue tip up: Tongue tip, narrowly grooved, contacts alveolar ridge behind *upper* incisors. Breath is continuously directed through narrow aperture between alveolar ridge and grooved tongue tip, creating turbulence. Tongue tip down: Tip of tongue contacts alveolar ridge behind *lower* incisors. Front of tongue, slightly grooved, is raised toward alveolar ridge and forms a narrow aperture through which breath is continuously directed against front teeth, creating turbulence. Lips are apart and neutral; may be in position for following vowel.
Voicing/Velopharyngeal Port	**Spelling Variations**
Voiceless—vocal folds *ab*duct. VP port is closed.	Variable spelling Pronounced as /z/ in busines*s*, /ʒ/ in treasure, /ʃ/ as in *s*ure x /ks/ as in wa*x*, fi*x* c as /s/ sound in *c*ity, *c*ycle sc *sc*epter, *sc*ene st with silent /t/ as in glis*t*en, tres*t*le ps silent /p/ as in *p*sychology s as plural form, present tense, or possessive, after voiceless consonant as in cape*s*, sit*s*, Pat'*s*
Word Position	**Clinical Information**
Initial, medial, and final positions in SAE	This phoneme is frequently misarticulated. One of the most frequently occurring consonants in SAE Common substitutions include /t/ /d/ or /ʃ/. Interdental lisp: substituted with /θ/ (tip of tongue protrudes between teeth) Lateral lisp: airflow *around* tongue rather than through front of oral cavity Cognate of /z/

/z/

Transcription Exercise 6–7   **Track: (CD 1, Track 34)**

		I	M	F
1.	kids			✗
2.	czar	✗		
3.	cheese			✗
4.	observe		✗	
5.	business		✗	
6.	nasal		✗	
7.	present		✗	
8.	is			✗
9.	seizure			
10.	bobsleds			✗

Transcription Exercise 6–8
Consonant: /z/

 Track: (CD 1, Track 35)
Refer to Study Card: 8

Phonetic Symbol	Target Word	Transcription
/z/	1. busy	bɪzi
	2. visit	vɪzɪt
	3. zircon	zɝkɑn
	4. weasel	wizɪl
	5. seas	siz
	6. zinnia	zinijə
	7. those	ðoz
	8. zucchini	zukini
	9. gives	givz

/z/

Distinctive Features	Tongue Position
Lingua-alveolar fricative Voiced, front, nonlabial, nonsonorant, continuant, sibilant, non-nasal / z / ⟶	See /s/ for description of production.

Voicing/Velopharyngeal Port	Spelling Variations
Voiced—vocal folds *ad*duct. VP port is closed.	s as in hi*s*, wa*s*, de*s*ign, *s*ci*s*sor*s* es plural forms or possessive as in kiss*es*, boy'*s* ss occurs as /z/ in sci*ss*ors sth a*sth*ma x *x*ylophone x forms /gz/ in e*x*amine [ɛgzæmɪn]

Word Position	Clinical Information
Initial, medial, and final positions in SAE	Commonly substituted with /d/ or /t/. Can also be produced as interdental or lateral lisp (see /s/ Clinical Information). Cognate of /s/

CAN YOU HEAR THE DIFFERENCE BETWEEN /s/ AND /z/?

Listening Exercise Final /z/   **Track: (CD 1, Track 36)**

It is not always easy to *hear* the difference between /s/ and /z/, especially in the final position of words. As you listen to the CD, pay attention to the /z/. The /z/ is emphasized in these words:

1. phase	16. news
2. cheese	17. sees
3. surprise	18. pies
4. fleas	19. rituals
5. tease	20. bruise
6. was	21. Eloise
7. tragedies	22. joys
8. wise	23. cardinals
9. rose	24. Japanese
10. bananas	25. is
11. cruise	26. tomatoes
12. eyes	27. skis
13. glows	28. kneels
14. choose	29. stereos
15. goes	30. advertise

Crossword Puzzle for /s/ and /z/

Answers in Appendix B

Directions: Transcribe the following words:

Across:

3. zip

4. sizzle

5. soldier

Down:

1. soups

2. zeal

3. Zorro

5. seasons

THE CENTER RING

Word Search #6

Answers in Appendix B

```
æ  h  m  s  t  o  ɑ  g  ɪ  t  m  k
k  æ  ɛ  l  ə  f  ɪ  n  t  s  z  ɑ
r  m  t  i  ɚ  r  h  d  r  k  ɛ  s
o  h  p  s  ɛ  ks aɪ t  m  ɛ  n  t
b  u  ɛ  ə  m  i  d  r  ɛ  o  tʃ u
æ  t  r  m  ɛ  ə  h  æ  k  r  ə  m
t  b  i  s  m  l  aʊ p  i  n  i  z
s  ɝ  k  ə  s  d  r  i  t  p  ɑ  l
j  ɑ  h  ɪ  k  e  g  z  i  b  r  ə
h  ð  æ  r  l  l  e  e  u  o  k  ɑ
u  k  l  k  aʊ e  t  aɪ g  ɚ  z  r
p  æ  o  n  n  b  d  dʒ d  t  o  z
s  t  w  l  z  n  ɔ  ɝ  i  e  t  i
s  l  aɪ ə  n  z  r  t  ɛ  n  t  s
```

Directions: Find and circle the words listed below which contain the /s/ or /z/ phonemes.

circus	clowns	acrobats
trapeze	zebra	lions
costumes	excitement	elephants
tigers	hoops	tents

Transcription Exercise 6–9
Fricative Consonants: / f / v / s / z /

 Track: (CD 1, Track 37)
Phoneme Study Cards: 7–10

1. festive ___festɪv___

2. Swiss ___swɪs___

3. vessel ___vɛsəl___

4. fanciful ___fænsɪfʊl___

5. measles ___mizəlz___

6. zest ___zɛst___

7. vivid ___vɪvɪd___

8. expensive ___ɛkspɛnsɪv___

9. businesses ___bɪznɪsɪz___

10. forgive ___fɔrgɪv___

11. soapsuds ___sopsʌdz___

12. fasten ___fæsɪn___

13. squeeze ___skwiz___

14. scissors ___sɪzɚz___

15. pharmacy ___farməsi___

16. Stephen ___stivɪn___

17. vice ___vɑɪs___

18. Switzerland ___swɪtzɚˈlænd___

19. safety ___sefti___

20. civilian ___sɪvɪljən___

/θ/

Transcription Exercise 6–10   **Track: (CD 1, Track 38)**

		I	M	F
1.	enthusiast		✗	
2.	Thursday	✗		
3.	thither	✗		
4.	Elizabeth			✗
5.	thirty-third	✗	✗	
6.	Gothic		✗	
7.	cathedral		✗	
8.	through	✗		
9.	anesthesia		✗	
10.	zenith			✗

Transcription Exercise 6–11
Consonant: /θ/

 Track: (CD 1, Track 39)
Refer to Study Card: 11

Phonetic Symbol	Target Word	Transcription
/θ/	1. thin	θɪn
	2. birthday	bɝθde
	3. width	wɪdθ
	4. teeth	tiθ
	5. throw	θro
	6. anything	ɪniθɪŋ
	7. north	norθ
	8. nothing	nʌθɪŋ
	9. thaw	θɔ

ðʌ

/θ/

Distinctive Features	Tongue Position
Interdental fricative Voiceless, front, nonlabial, nonsonorant, continuant, nonsibilant, non-nasal /θ/ ⟶	Sides of tongue are against upper molars. Tip and blade of tongue are spread wide and thin in space between teeth. Breath is continuously emitted between front teeth. Lips are apart and neutral.

Voicing/Velopharyngeal Port	Spelling Variations
Voiceless—vocal folds *ab*duct. VP port is closed.	th is the only spelling th ba*th*, mon*th* th some*th*ing, au*th*or thr *thr*ee

Word Positions	Clinical Information
Initial, medial, and final positions in SAE	Also known as "theta" A sound unique to the English language (Edwards, 2003) Commonly substituted with /t/s/f/ Cognate of /ð/

/ð/

Transcription Exercise 6–12   **Track: (CD 1, Track 40)**

		I	M	F
1.	them	✗		
2.	clothe			✗
3.	Heather		✗	
4.	rhythm		✗	
5.	teeth			
6.	north			
7.	whether		✗	
8.	thigh			
9.	northern		✗	
10.	weather		✗	

Transcription Exercise 6–13
Consonant: /ð/

 Track: (CD 1, Track 41)
Refer to Study Card: 12

Phonetic Symbol	Target Word	Transcription
/ð/	1. this	ðɪs
	2. either	iðɚ
	3. there	ðɛr
	4. father	faðɚ
	5. seethe	siθ
	6. though	ðo
	7. mother	mʌðɚ
	8. teethe	tið
	9. smooth	smuð

/ð/

Distinctive Features	Tongue Position
Interdental fricative Voiced front, nonlabial, nonsonorant, continuant, nonsibilant, non-nasal /ð/ →	Same tongue position as for production of /θ/

Voicing/Velopharyngeal Port	Spelling Variations
Voiced—vocal folds *ad*ducted. VP port is closed.	th is the only spelling th occurs in frequently used words such as *the, this, that, they, them, then, these, there, those* th ba*the*, soo*the*, bo*ther*, fea*ther*

Word Positions	Clinical Information
Initial, medial, and final positions in SAE	A sound unique to the English language (Edwards, 2003) Commonly substituted with /d/ and /t/ Cognate of /θ/

Transcription Exercise 6–14   **Track: (CD 1, Track 42)**

It is often difficult for beginning phonetics students to hear the difference between the voiced "th" /ð/ and unvoiced "th"/θ/. It can be helpful if you say words with these phonemes to "feel" the difference. When you pronounce the voiced "th," you will feel a vibration produced by the tongue placement between the central incisors. In addition, the vocal folds vibrate. Contrast this production with the unvoiced "th" in which there is no vocal fold vibration. Directions: Say each word and write the symbol for the voiced /ð/ or unvoiced /θ/ phoneme. Listen to the CD if you need help.

1. wreathe (verb) ð		16. thank θ
2. than ð		17. although ð
3. earthworm θ		18. thou ð
4. bath θ		19. rhythm ð
5. ungathered ð		20. pathway θ
6. seethe ð		21. Judith θ
7. stethoscope θ		22. healthy θ
8. blithe ð		23. marathon θ
9. amethyst θ		24. together ð
10. featherbed ð		25. thump θ
11. weatherman ð		26. Southerner ð
12. locksmith θ		27. these ð
13. with θ		28. either ð
14. though ð		29. lather ð
15. either ð		30. Keith θ

Crossword Puzzle for /θ/ and /ð/

Answers in Appendix B

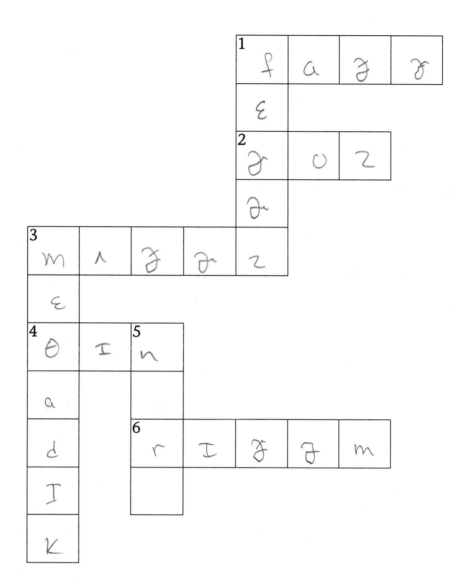

Directions: Transcribe the following words:

Across:

1. father
2. those
3. mothers
4. thin
6. rhythm

Down:

1. feathers
3. methodic
5. north

INTERDENTAL FRICATIVE

Word Search #7   Answers in Appendix B

g	t	k	ɛ	l	v	b	ʌ	k	b	m	s
ɝ	ʒ	p	æ	θ	h	e	b	m	ɛ	θ	aʊ
k	p	o	r	ɛ	e	ð	ɛ	ɪ	d	ð	d
l	p	θ	t	m	v	m	ɛ	o	e	æ	m
o	o	r	æ	ð	b	ɑ	ð	ɚ	l	n	ɑ
ð	k	ɛ	n	p	f	θ	l	d	t	t	m
e	θ	d	d	ə	n	ə	ð	ɚ	p	æ	æ
v	n	k	m	g	tʃ	æ	t	ə	k	n	θ
æ	ɚ	ð	g	r	θ	ɪ	ŋ	l	l	r	ɪ
θ	n	t	æ	ɝ	ɝ	θ	ɚ	z	ɑ	t	ɛ
r	g	n	ð	v	d	r	w	ɪ	θ	aʊ	t
j	b	o	ɚ	k	h	ɪ	b	s	e	t	i
ə	æ	g	m	s	aʊ	θ	ɑ	l	m	ɛ	g
t	θ	t	θ	p	z	n	r	i	æ	n	k

Directions: Find and circle the words listed below which contain the /θ/ or /ð/ phonemes.

thread	moth	than	cloth
third	without	bother	clothe
thing	math	bath	path
south	another	bathe	gather

Transcription Exercise 6–15
Interdental Consonants: / θ / ð /

 Track: (CD 1, Track 43)
Phoneme Study Cards: 11–12

1. bike-a-thon   baɪk-ʌ-θɔn

2. Wadsworth   wadɹwɝθ

3. southeastern   saʊθistɚn

4. arithmetic   ʌrɪθmʌtɪk

5. seventeenth   sɛvʌntinθ

6. threaten   θrɛtɪn

7. undergrowth   ʌndɚgroθ

8. southernmost   sʌðɚnmost

9. Thunderbird   θʌndɚbɝd

10. Plymouth   plɪmʌθ

11. ruthlessly   ruθlɛsli

12. Witherspoon   wɪðɚspun

13. heartthrob   hartθrab

14. worthy   wɝði

15. thriving   θraɪvɪn

16. another   ðnʌðɚ

17. methodic   mɛθadɪk

18. thoughtless   θaʔlɛs

19. hundredth   hʌndrɛθ

20. leather   lɛðɚ

/h/

Transcription Exercise 6–16 **Track: (CD 1, Track 44)**

		I	M	F
1.	whom	X		
2.	rehearse		X	
3.	hitchhike	X	X	
4.	unwholesome		X	
5.	Jose	X		
6.	inhale		X	
7.	gila monster	X		
8.	habitat	X		
9.	mahogany		X	
10.	exhalation		X

Transcription Exercise 6–17
Consonant: /h/

 Track: (CD 1, Track 45)
Refer to Study Card: 15

Phonetic Symbol	Target Word	Transcription
/h/	1. heft	hɛft
	2. harbor	harbɚ
	3. mohair	mohɛr
	4. uphill	ʌphɪl
	5. hum	hʌm
	6. inherit	ɪnhɛrɪt
	7. rehearse	rihɚs
	8. hermit	hɝmɪt
	9. unhook	ʌnhʊk

/h/

Distinctive Features	Tongue Position ✓
Glottal fricative Voiceless, back, nonlabial, nonsonorant, continuant, nonsibilant, non-nasal 	No consistent articulatory pattern. Tongue and lips are in position for following phoneme. Turbulence is created at level of glottis. Breath is directed through the oral cavity.

Voicing/Velopharyngeal Port	Spelling Variations
If produced in isolation, /h/ is voiceless—vocal folds are *ab*ducted. VP port is closed.	wh *wh*om, *wh*ole gh silent as in Hu*gh* h silent in *h*onor, *h*onest

Word Positions	Clinical Information
Initial and medial positions in SAE	May be replaced with glottal stop in certain dialects

/hw/ or /ʍ/

Transcription Exercise 6–18   🄲 **Track: (CD 1, Track 46)**

		I	M	F
1.	wheel	✗		
2.	queen		✗	
3.	swear		✗	
4.	why	✗		
5.	suede		✗	
6.	where	✗		
7.	wholewheat		✗	
8.	wear			
9.	wagon			
10.	square		✗	

Note: Although use of this phoneme is not common, it is helpful for purposes of "ear training" to discriminate between /hw/ and /w/. With the exception of "wear" and "wagon," the remainder of the words in this exercise can be produced with /hw/ as an alternative pronunciation.

Transcription Exercise 6–19
Consonant: /hw/ also /ʍ/

 Track: (CD 1, Track 47)
Refer to Study Card: 16

Phonetic Symbol	Target Word	Transcription
/hw/	1. whim	ʍɪm
	2. overwhelm	ovɚʍɛlm
	3. whip	ʍɪp
	4. twenty	tʍɛnti
	5. schwa	ʃʍa
	6. white	ʍaɪt
	7. somewhere	sʌmʍɛr
	8. whether	mɛʒɚ
	9. wharf	ʍorf

/hw/ or /ʍ/

Distinctive Features	Tongue Position
Labial-velar (bilabial) fricative Voiceless, nonsibilant, continuant 	Back of tongue may be raised toward soft palate, or may be in low back position for /h/. Lips may be rounded. Breath is directed through oral cavity and lip opening.

Voicing/Velopharyngeal Port	Spelling Variations
Voiceless; however, vocal folds *add*uct slightly to create turbulence. VP port is closed.	w following /s/ as in s*w*im, s*w*ag; following /t/ as in t*w*ig, t*w*elve, and following "th" as in th*w*art, may be produced with the /ʍ/ wh *w*heel, some*w*here

Word Positions	Clinical Information
Initial and medial positions in SAE	Also called inverted "w" Most commonly produced as /w/

Transcription Exercise 6–20
Consonants: /h/hw/ or /ʍ/

 Track: (CD 1, Track 48)
Phoneme Study Cards: 15–16

1. hedgehog _____ hɛdʒhɑɡ _____

2. suede _____ sʍed _____

3. whirl _____ ʍɝl _____

4. whom _____ hʊm _____

5. sway _____ sʍe _____

6. wahoo _____ wɑhu _____

7. whine _____ ʍɑɪn _____

8. handshake _____ hænd ʃek _____

9. hair _____ bɛr _____

10. whiff _____ ʍɪf _____

11. who _____ hu _____

12. whammy _____ ʍæmɪ _____

13. wholehearted _____ holhɑrtɪd _____

14. where _____ ʍɛr _____

15. pinwheel _____ pɪnʍil _____

16. hymn _____ hɪm _____

17. persuade _____ pɝsʍed _____

18. whistle _____ ʍɪsʒl _____

19. Ohio _____ ohɑɪo _____

20. whose _____ huz _____

/ʃ/

Transcription Exercise 6–21   **Track: (CD 1, Track 49)**

		I	M	F
1.	condition		✕	
2.	usher		✕	
3.	tissue		✕	
4.	brochure		✕	
5.	chiffon	✕		
6.	initial		✕	
7.	treasure			
8.	licorice			✕
9.	creation		✕	
10.	shoebrush	✕		✕

Transcription Exercise 6–22
Consonant: /ʃ/

 Track: (CD 1, Track 50)
Refer to Study Card: 13

Phonetic Symbol	Target Word	Transcription
/ʃ/	1. shoe	ʃu
	2. mustache	mʌstæʃ
	3. ocean	oʃən
	4. insure	ɪnʃɚ
	5. wish	wɪʃ
	6. ship	ʃɪp
	7. relish	rɛlɪf
	8. shake	ʃek
	9. fashion	fæʃən

/ʃ/

Distinctive Features	Articulatory Production
Lingua-palatal fricative Voiceless, back, nonsonorant, continuant, sibilant, non-nasal	Sides of tongue contact upper molars. Tip of tongue is at the lower central incisors; front of tongue raised toward hard palate. Breathstream is directed through and against slightly opened front teeth to create audible friction. Lips are slightly rounded and protruded, approximating position for /ʊ/.

Voicing/Velopharyngeal Port	Spelling Variations
Voiceless—vocal folds *ab*duct. VP port is closed.	s *s*ugar, in*s*urance c o*c*ean ch *ch*ic, musta*ch*e tion na*tion*, ac*tion* sc con*sc*ience chs fu*chs*ia

Word Positions	Clinical Information
Initial, medial, and final positions in SAE	Common articulatory substitution: t/ʃ, d/ʃ, s/ʃ Cognate of /ʒ/

/ʒ/

Transcription Exercise 6–23   Track: (CD 1, Track 51)

		I	M	F
1.	vision		✗	
2.	aphasia		✗	
3.	garage			✗
4.	station			
5.	treasure		✗	
6.	Persia		✗	
7.	closure		✗	
8.	rouge			✗
9.	composure		✗	
10.	television		✗	

Note: #3, garage, may also be produced as [gʌrɑdʒ].

Transcription Exercise 6–24
Consonant: /ʒ/

 Track: (CD 1, Track 52)
Refer to Study Card: 14

Phonetic Symbol	Target Word	Transcription
/ʒ/	1. regime	rɛʒim
	2. loge	loʒ
	3. pleasure	plɛʒɚ
	4. division	dɪvɪʒɪn
	5. usual	juʒuəl
	6. collision	k
	7. beige	beʒ
	8. collage	kolɑʒ
	9. casual	kæsuəl

/ʒ/

Distinctive Features	Tongue Position
Lingua-palatal fricative Voiced, back, nonlabial, nonsonorant, continuant, sibilant, non-nasal 	See /ʃ/ for description of production.

Voicing/Velopharyngeal Port	Spelling Variations
Voiced—vocal folds *ad*duct. VP port is closed.	s as in mea*s*ure, occa*s*ion g(e) bei*ge*, presti*ge* z a*z*ure, sei*z*ure

Word Positions	Clinical Information
Medial and final positions in SAE	Common articulation error is substitution of /d/, /t/ and omission Cognate of /ʃ/

Crossword Puzzle for /ʃ/ and /ʒ/

Answers in Appendix B

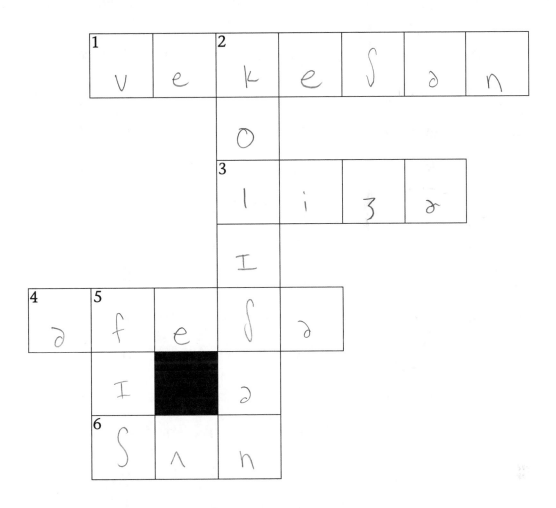

Directions: Transcribe the following words:

Across:
1. vacation
3. leisure
4. aphasia
6. shun

Down:
2. collision
5. fish

UNDER THE SEA

Word Search #8

Answers in Appendix B

```
ʃ  æ  l  o  k  ʃ  s  z  n  æ  aɪ p
d  d  d  p  r  r  ɪ  ɪ  k  n  g  ɔ
ɪ  l  ʌ  æ  o  ɪ  t  k  θ  o  l  l
k  n  k  n  j  m  i  l  ɪ  ʃ  k  ə
d  r  m  ʃ  ɪ  p  s  s  ŋ  ə  r  n
ɪ  ɑ  ə  d  u  r  m  l  s  n  ɑ  i
s  d  ɪ  s  n  o  ə  z  z  d  f  ʒ
n  s  n  d  t  f  ɪ  ʃ  k  r  ɝ  ə
ʃ  o  l  e  θ  e  ð  ɔ  o  u  j  k
i  m  m  l  w  z  ʃ  ə  l  ʃ  æ  d
ʃ  ɑ  r  k  d  i  l  ə  h  w  b  o
l  i  s  p  r  o  n  ð  n  ɛ  r  l
æ  t  r  ɛ  ʒ  ɚ  tʃ ɛ  s  t  t  æ
p  m  k  l  æ  m  ʃ  ɛ  l  b  m  b
h  ɪ  tʃ u  o  d  ɔ  ə  s  ɚ  ɪ  ʒ
d  k  ɪ  z  b  ʌ  r  l  ɛ  m  n  r
```

Directions: Find and circle the words listed below which contain the /ʃ/ or /ʒ/ phonemes.

shrimp	treasure chest	shallow	ships
shore	crustacean	shark	fish
clamshell	ocean	shoal	shad
Polynesia			

STUDY QUESTIONS

1. Why are the /h/ and /hw/ classified as fricatives but are not cognates?

_____

_____

2. What is the source of friction for for /h/ and /hw/?

_____

_____

3. What is the tongue position for production of /f/ and /v/?

_____

_____

4. What are two ways the /s/ and /z/ can be produced?

_____

_____

5. What is the difference between an interdental lisp and a lateral lisp?

_____

_____

6. What is the Greek name for the voiceless "th"?

_____

_____

7. What is the tongue position for production of /ʃ/ and /ʒ/?

_____

_____

CHAPTER

7

Consonants: Affricates /tʃ/dʒ/

Learning Objectives

After reading this chapter, you will be able to:

1. Describe how affricates are produced.

2. Identify manner of production of affricates.

3. Explain how to correctly write the two components of the affricates.

4. List spelling variations for the affricates.

5. Transcribe words using affricate consonants.

The affricates are a combination of a stop-consonant immediately followed by a fricative, produced in the same breath. They are also called "stop-fricatives," which describes their manner of production. Affricates are considered obstruents as they are produced with an obstructed breath stream.

Some phoneticians prefer to write the two components of the affricates touching each other to emphasize that they are produced with a single breath impulse and to eliminate confusing the symbols with two separate phonemes.

/tʃ/

Transcription Exercise 7–1

Track: (CD 1, Track 53)

		I	M	F
1.	chef			
2.	hatchet		✓	
3.	pitch			✓
4.	brochure			
5.	chord			
6.	culture		✓	
7.	ache			
8.	machine			
9.	church	✓		
10.	future		✓	

Transcription Exercise 7–2
Consonant: /tʃ/

 Track: (CD 1, Track 54)
Refer to Study Card: 17

Phonetic Symbol	Target Word	Transcription
/tʃ/	1. chin	
	2. peaches	
	3. which	
	4. cheese	
	5. lunch	
	6. teacher	
	7. children	
	8. scotch	
	9. furniture	

/tʃ/

Distinctive Features	Tongue Position
Alveopalatal affricate Voiceless, back, nonlabial, nonsonorant, noncontinuant, sibilant, non-nasal / tʃ /	Sides of tongue against upper molars. Tip and blade of tongue close on or just behind upper alveolar ridge. Air held and compressed in oral cavity; exploded as audible breath through broad opening between alveolar ridge and front of tongue. Turbulence is created. Lips are apart and neutral. The phoneme begins as a stop /t/ with tongue moving into position for /ʃ/.

Voicing/Velopharyngeal Port	Spelling Variations
Voiceless—vocal folds *ab*duct. VP port is closed.	tch ma*tch*, ca*tch* t(ure) frac*ture*, furni*ture* t(ion) men*tion*, ques*tion* nsion with intruded /t/ for /ntʃ/ as in te*nsion* [tɛntʃən] t(u) vir*tue*, na*tural* Infrequently with c as in *cello*

Word Position	Clinical Information
Initial, medial, and final positions in SAE	Common articulation error of substitution of /t/ or /d/ or omitted Cognate of /dʒ/

/dʒ/

Transcription Exercise 7–3   **Track: (CD 1, Track 55)**

		I	M	F
1.	garage			✓
2.	budget		✓	
3.	ginger		✓	
4.	dungeon		✓	
5.	jump	✓		
6.	education		✓	
7.	gesture	✓		
8.	voyage			✓
9.	engine		✓	
10.	splurge			✓

Transcription Exercise 7–4
Consonant: /dʒ/

 Track: (CD 1, Track 56)
Refer to Study Card: 18

Phonetic Symbol	Target Word	Transcription
/dʒ/	1. junk	
	2. enjoy	
	3. urged	
	4. vigil	
	5. wage	
	6. gem	
	7. jumbo	
	8. collagen	
	9. fudge	

/dʒ/

Distinctive Features	Tongue Position
Alveopalatal affricate Voiced, back, nonlabial, nonsonorant, noncontinuant, sibilant, non-nasal 	See /tʃ/ for production. This phoneme begins as a stop /d/ with tongue moving into position for /ʒ/.

Voicing/Velopharyngeal Port	Spelling Variations
Voiced—vocal folds *ad*duct. VP port is closed.	gg exa*gg*erate d cor*d*ial, gra*d*ual j *j*uice, *j*erk dge e*dge* g tra*g*ic, en*g*ine, *g*ypsy dj a*dj*ust

Word Position	Clinical Information
Initial, medial, and final positions in SAE	Cognate of /tʃ/

Crossword Puzzle for /tʃ/ and /dʒ/

Answers in Appendix B

Directions: Transcribe the following words:

Across:

2. angels

3. rejoice

5. preachers

Down:

1. clergy

4. psalms

AFFRICATES

Word Search #9

Answers in Appendix B

```
k  p  ɑ  s  s  ɑ  g  e  z  e  dʒ i  p  b  r  j  m  ɛ
n  k  w  tʃ k  v  u  i  tʃ kʍ o  f  z  g  j  r  s  n
d  b  t  s  i  ə  b  ɛ  ks tʃ e  n  dʒ n  u  tʃ v  d
j  s  p  k  æ  z  h  v  s  t  o  h  i  g  m  v  ɪ  z
m  j  æ  h  u  h  ɑ  h  w  n  ɛ  w  f  dʒ p  r  l  t
p  æ  d  v  ɛ  n  tʃ ɚ  k  θ  u  p  ʌ  z  s  p  ɪ  m
m  e  o  z  v  l  ɝ  p  æ  s  ɪ  dʒ ɛ  p  o  k  dʒ n
m  m  s  h  p  b  f  o  g  s  t  ʃ  dʒ h  w  g  g  ŋ
g  ɑ  dʒ ɪ  ŋ  k  s  s  t  z  æ  l  ɪ  o  e  æ  ʌ  ɑ
t  v  ɪ  f  k  g  θ  ɔ  d  ʃ  l  k  u  j  h  s  u  ʍ
v  d  l  i  æ  o  n  d  dʒ h  l  m  f  v  ʌ  ə  j
t  f  ɛ  r  ʌ  i  ʒ  r  n  ʒ  f  æ  æ  z  f  n  s  r
r  b  r  ɪ  dʒ ɛ  z  l  ɪ  m  z  dʒ p  ɛ  ɪ  b  z  l
j  b  w  e  ɪ  f  ŋ  ɪ  l  n  m  ɪ  v  ks h  i  ʃ  ʌ
i  w  o  o  k  v  ɛ  ʊ  æ  ŋ  d  k  m  u  w  tʃ h  ɛ
l  n  h  r  ʃ  ð  e  ɚ  tʃ ɔ  o  v  h  n  j  p  ʒ  p
ʊ  z  s  ɪ  n  tʃ ə  p  f  o  s  p  ɛ  h  t  i  tʃ t
z  h  t  u  t  h  ʍ b  v  u  n  ʒ  l  m  r  w  dʒ d
```

Directions: Find and circle the words below which contain the /tʃ/ and /dʒ/ phonemes.

cheese	jinks	age	cinch
challenge	judge	adventure	village
exchange	magic	passage	
beach	bridges	teach	

Transcription Exercise 7–5
Fricative and Affricate Consonants: /ʃ/ʒ/tʃ/dʒ/

Track (CD 1, Track 57)
Phoneme Study Cards: 13–14, 17–18

1. shoeshine   _____

2. digestion   _____

3. confusion   _____

4. entourage   _____

5. agriculture   _____

6. vivacious   _____

7. sabotage   _____

8. enchanted   _____

9. Jake   _____

10. ship-to-shore   _____

11. stagecoach   _____

12. childish   _____

13. hodgepodge   _____

14. Parisian   _____

15. suggestion   _____

16. chinchilla   _____

17. collection   _____

18. fortunate   _____

19. beautician   _____

20. visualize   _____

STUDY QUESTIONS

1. What symbols combine to form affricates?

_____

_____

2. Affricates are also called:

_____

_____

3. Why are affricates considered obstruents?

_____

_____

4. What is a common articulatory substitution for /tʃ/?

_____

_____

5. List two words that contain the /tʃ/ and /dʒ/ phonemes.

_____

_____

6. Why is it important to have the two components of affricates touch?

_____

_____

8

Consonants:
Oral Resonants /w/j/l/r/

Learning Objectives

After reading this chapter, you will be able to:

1. Define the term "approximation" and relationship to oral resonant production.

2. State which oral resonant can intrude between two vowels.

3. Describe unique airflow for production of /l/.

4. State how preceding vowels can influence /r/ production.

5. Transcribe words using oral resonant consonants.

Unlike the stop-consonants or fricatives, which are produced with full or partial obstruction of the vocal tract, the /w/j/l/ and /r/ consonants are vowel-like, as the breathstream glides smoothly through the vocal tract. The obstruction that occurs with this group of consonants is caused by *approximation* of the articulators. Approximation is defined as a position of closeness of the articulators.

The /r/ and /l/ phonemes are also referred to as *liquids*. However, most phoneticians view /r/ as a glide. These consonants are termed *oral resonant* due to changes in the oral cavity. These changes result from raising or lowering the mandible, lowering or elevating the tongue, and changing lip opening and rounding of the lips. All of these can change the shape of the oral cavity.

/w/

Transcription Exercise 8–1   Track: (CD 1, Track 58)

		I	M	F
1.	once	✓		
2.	widow	✓		
3.	Guam		✓	
4.	twice		✓	
5.	iguana		✓	
6.	where	✓		
7.	kiwi		✓	
8.	question		✓	
9.	willow	✓		
10.	anguish		✓	

Transcription Exercise 8–2
Consonant: /w/

 Track: (CD 1, Track 59)
Refer to Study Card: 25

Phonetic Symbol	Target Word	Transcription
/w/	1. wax	
	2. jaguar	
	3. beware	
	4. swell	
	5. wonder	
	6. queen	
	7. forward	
	8. twin	
	9. wet	

/w/

Distinctive Features	Tongue Position
Bilabial lingua-palatal or lingua-velar glide Voiced, back, labial, sonorant, noncontinuant, nonsibilant, non-nasal 	High back position (as for /u/). Moves into position for following sound. Lips rounded and protruded, but may unround quickly for transition to next sound.

Voicing/Velopharyngeal Port	Spelling Variations
Voiced—vocal folds *ad*ducted. VP port is closed.	o *one, once, everyone* w silent in *who, whole, sword, answer, write* (ng) u /w/ glide occurs for /u/ in *language* [læŋgwɪdʒ]

Word Positions	Clinical Information
Initial and medial positions in SAE	kw represents the "q" sound as in *quit* Can be omitted from clusters such as sw in *sweet*

ORAL RESONANTS

Word Search #10   Answers in Appendix B

g	w	ɑ	n	t	ɑ	n	ɑ	m	o	b	e
ʃ	ɛ	w	e	r	s	ð	r	d	b	ʃ	s
s	ɑ	b	s	ð	ŋ	l	r	j	o	m	h
æ	p	v	ɪ	v	o	ʃ	tʃ	b	m	n	aʊ
n	ɑ	k	v	f	w	ɑ	t	ɚ	l	u	w
w	p	r	ɪ	i	ʌ	ə	j	v	w	θ	ɪ
ɑ	w	ɝ	l	d	w	ɔ	r	w	ʌ	n	t
n	tʃ	ɪ	w	p	b	t	d	k	g	s	z
h	ɑ	b	ɔ	r	æ	p	e	p	k	w	ɚ
ɪ	ʒ	n	r	e	dʒ	ɚ	u	ɔ	o	θ	o
l	ʃ	æ	ʊ	t	b	n	z	b	l	ɑ	ð
r	w	ɛ	p	ə	n	e	w	l	d	j	ɝ
d	p	ɛ	t	e	v	i	h	b	w	e	m
p	æ	n	d	p	aʊ	w	ɚ	ʊ	ɔ	l	u
ɚ	z	d	ɔ	l	t	r	d	ʒ	r	v	i

Directions: Find and circle the words listed below which contain the /w/ phoneme.

Civil War	howitzer
World War One	Cold War
Guantanamo Bay	power
Waterloo	weapon

/j/

Transcription. Exercise 8–3　　　　　　　　　　**Track: (CD 1, Track 60)**

		I	M	F
1.	inject			
2.	royal		✓	
3.	yet	✓		
4.	zillion		✓	
5.	bunion		✓	
6.	spaniel			
7.	yoyo	✓	✓	
8.	layette		✓	
9.	figure		✓	
10.	coyote		✓	

Transcription Exercise 8–4
Consonant: /j/

 Track: (CD 1, Track 61)
Refer to Study Card: 23

Phonetic Symbol	Target Word	Transcription
/j/	1. your	
	2. beyond	
	3. yield	
	4. papaya	
	5. yonder	
	6. familiar	
	7. yarn	
	8. billion	
	9. yes	

/j/

Distinctive Features	Tongue Position
Lingua-palatal glide Voiced, back, nonlabial, sonorant, noncontinuant, nonsibilant, non-nasal 	Tongue is in high front position, approximating /i/ and is ready to move into position for the next sound.

Voicing/Velopharyngeal Port	Spelling Variations
Voiced—vocal folds *ad*duct. VP port is closed.	i on*i*on, Will*i*am j hallelu*j*ah l bouil*l*on /j/ is often intrusive between words ending in /i/ or /ɪ/ and those beginning with a vowel: see it [sijɪt]

Word Positions	Clinical Information
Initial and medial positions in SAE	Articulation error: substituted with /w/ or omitted

/l/

Transcription Exercise 8–5   **Track: (CD 1, Track 62)**

		I	M	F
1.	mall			✓
2.	linoleum	✓	✓	
3.	whale			✓
4.	apple			✓
5.	fellow		✓	
6.	calves			
7.	lullaby	✓	✓	
8.	flotilla			
9.	helm		✓	
10.	sociable			✓

Transcription Exercise 8–6
Consonant: /l/

 Track: (CD 1, Track 63)
Refer to Study Card: 22

Phonetic Symbol	Target Word	Transcription
/l/	1. lucky	
	2. lemon	
	3. clown	
	4. sandal	
	5. golden	
	6. else	
	7. bridal	
	8. flea	
	9. Leon	

/l/

Distinctive Features	Tongue Position
Lingua-alveolar lateral (liquid) Voiced, front, nonlabial, sonorant, noncontinuant, nonsibilant, non-nasal /l/ →	Tip of tongue and part of blade contact upper alveolar ridge. Lips are apart and neutral. Airflow is around the sides of the tongue for lateral emission of airstream.
Voicing/Velopharyngeal Port	**Spelling Variations**
Voiced—vocal folds *ad*duct. VP port is closed.	Appears consistently as *l* le bott*le*, midd*le* el funn*el*, kenn*el* sl with silent *s* in ai*sl*e
Word Positions	**Clinical Information**
Initial, medial, and final positions in SAE	This phoneme's unique feature is the airflow around the *sides* of the tongue.

/r/

Transcription Exercise 8–7   Track: (CD 1, Track 64)

		I	M	F
1.	wrap	✓		
2.	rye	✓		
3.	scar			✓
4.	report	✓	✓	
5.	rubber	✓		
6.	wardrobe		✓	
7.	wry	✓		
8.	garden		✓	
9.	before			✓
10.	deer			✓

Transcription Exercise 8–8
Consonant: /r/

 Track: (CD 1, Track 65)
Refer to Study Card: 24

Phonetic Symbol	Target Word	Transcription
/r/	1. write	
	2. impress	
	3. reduce	
	4. sorry	
	5. rhyme	
	6. already	
	7. chair	
	8. rub	
	9. bar	

/r/

Distinctive Features	Tongue Position
Alveo-palatal liquid (glide) Voiced, front, labial, sonorant, noncontinuant, nonsibilant, non-nasal ← /r/	Sides of the tongue are against upper molars. Back of tongue may be slightly elevated. Front of tongue usually is in close approximation to alveolar ridge. Retroflex position: Produced as above but tongue tip curls up and back. Lips may be slightly protruded similar to /ʊ/ but usually take the position of the surrounding vowel. If tongue tip is curled back toward palate, referred to as retroflex.

Voicing/Velopharyngeal Port	Spelling Variations
Voiced—vocal folds *ad*duct. VP port is closed.	wr *wr*ote, *wr*en rh *rh*inoceros, *rh*yme

Word Positions	Clinical Information
Initial, medial, and final positions in SAE	Common articulation error is substitution of w/r, especially in children under the age of 7 years. The IPA cites /ɹ/ but phoneticians in the USA use /r/.

Influence of the /r/ Sound

The /r/ phoneme can influence the vowel which precedes it. The vowels /i/ɛ/ɑ/o/ can occur with the /r/ in the same syllable as in the words "deer" [dir], "care [kɛr], "star" [stɑr], and "more" [mor].

The influence of the /r/ sound occurs especially in the vowel + r combination of /ɛr/ as in the word "hair" [hɛr]. Because of the location of the vowel adjacent to the /r/, the front of the tongue is in a lower position than would normally be expected. In this way, the tongue position makes the vowel sound of the /e/ closer to that of /ɛ/, resulting in the use of /ɛr/.

/ir/

Transcription Exercise 8–9

Track: (CD 1, Track 66)

		I	M	F
1.	spear			
2.	weird			
3.	series			
4.	steer			
5.	pear			
6.	fierce			
7.	era			
8.	career			
9.	mirth			
10.	wire			

/ɛr/

Transcription Exercise 8–10   **Track: (CD 1, Track 67)**

		I	M	F
1.	stair			
2.	square			
3.	barrel			
4.	ware			
5.	trailer			
6.	stare			
7.	pearl			
8.	chair			
9.	bear			
10.	caramel			

/ɑr/

Transcription Exercise 8–11   **Track: (CD 1, Track 68)**

		I	M	F
1.	heart			
2.	star			
3.	sergeant			
4.	farce			
5.	carriage			
6.	stare			
7.	marry			
8.	marine			
9.	party			
10.	carbon			

/or/

Transcription Exercise 8–12   **Track: (CD 1, Track 69)**

		I	M	F
1.	fourth			
2.	quart			
3.	parlor			
4.	wharf			
5.	soar			
6.	wart			
7.	rumor			
8.	court			
9.	pour			
10.	world			

VOWEL +r

Word Search #11

Answers in Appendix B

```
t    n    ʒ    g    f    o    r    s    k    o    r    m
k    p    s    ʃ    j    s    g    o    v    f    o    e
e    z    ə    ɪ    ʌ    j    i    r    l    i    ʒ    o
k    n    ɛ    u    g    ɑ    r    d    b    z    ɔ    f
r    ks   o    j    i    t    θ    h    m    θ    ʊ    i
ɛ    r    f    ɛ    r    r    d    f    m    ɝ    i    r
f    o    r    w    o    r    n    w    ɑ    ʌ    ɪ    s
b    g    k    ɛ    r    w    r    o    r    n    ɛ    p
u    s    r    p    e    ɝ    i    r    ʃ    ə    ð    b
l    k    tʃ   k    ɑ    r    f    ɛ    r    h    e    t
k    w    j    d    r    s    z    s    l    ɛ    d    d
ɛ    ɛ    z    s    n    m    ɑ    ŋ    dʒ   z    ɛ    k
ə    r    z    ɚ    k    o    r    t    j    ɑ    r    d
r    g    ʊ    p    o    r    z    ʊ    w    o    i    g
```

Directions: Find and circle the words listed below which contain the vowel + r sounds: /ir/or/ar/ɛr/.

yearly	guard	czars	dairy	forewarn
sword	square	carfare	pours	
ear	marsh	airfare	fourscore	
gear	fierce	careworn	courtyard	

Crossword Puzzle for /j/, /l/, and /r/

Answers in Appendix B

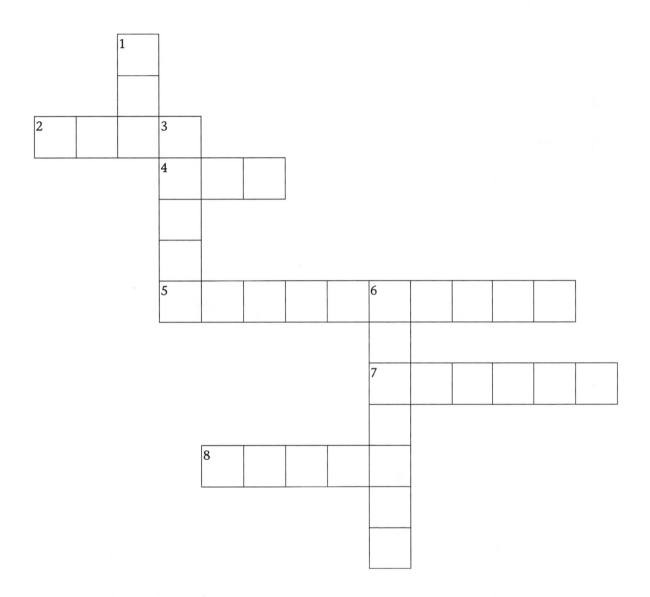

Directions: Transcribe the following words:

Across:
2. yellow
4. rose
5. jungle green
7. violet
8. maroon

Down:
1. teal
3. orange
6. lavender

WHAT'S IN A NAME?

Word Search #12   Answers in Appendix B

r	u	θ	v	g	e	h	k	o	w	k	l
s	ə	s	ɪ	o	k	a	l	i	n	m	o
ɪ	n	s	ɑ	g	n	j	u	k	r	v	r
l	r	r	ə	b	m	ŋ	i	o	ɝ	ɛ	ɛ
ɛ	ə	u	f	l	o	t	z	θ	ʌ	s	t
r	l	d	r	ə	s	ə	l	l	ɛ	o	ə
i	d	a	m	t	j	o	h	æ	n	r	ɚ
s	f	f	r	a	n	ə	l	d	ʃ	t	i
o	p	ks	k	d	e	r	u	ð	s	m	l
l	o	r	e	n	e	f	ə	t	s	r	e
t	t	dʒ	g	g	ʃ	o	ʊ	b	j	ɛ	n
m	ɪ	o	l	ɪ	v	i	ə	tʃ	ɝ	t	ð
r	h	r	z	ʒ	ð	ɔ	ɑ	ɪ	t	k	o
e	h	j	o	l	æ	n	d	ə	ɑ	w	ə

Directions: Find and circle the words listed below which contain the /j/, /l/, or /r/ phonemes.

Rudolph	Ronald	Ruth
Yolanda	Louise	Colleen
Russell	Johann	Elaine
Olivia	Loretta	Yetta
Lorraine	Larry	Rebecca

Transcription Exercise 8–13
Vowel + r: /or/ir/ɛr/ɑr/

 Track: (CD 1, Track 70)
Phoneme Study Cards: 44–47

1. earmark   _____

2. careworn   _____

3. ore   _____

4. spears   _____

5. carport   _____

6. sheer   _____

7. hardware   _____

8. dart   _____

9. forlorn   _____

10. rare   _____

11. sparse   _____

12. aardvark   _____

13. jeer   _____

14. bore   _____

15. foursquare   _____

16. farce   _____

17. coarse   _____

18. smears   _____

19. starch   _____

20. bear   _____

Transcription Exercise 8–14
Oral Resonant Consonants: /l/r/j/w/

 Track: (CD 1, Track 71)
Phoneme Study Cards: 22–25

1. yoke   _____

2. dwarf   _____

3. leeway   _____

4. dominion   _____

5. quibble   _____

6. larceny   _____

7. uranium   _____

8. illustrate   _____

9. rally   _____

10. Sawyer   _____

11. radiator   _____

12. quietly   _____

13. valiant   _____

14. frequency   _____

15. lawyer   _____

16. wayward   _____

17. Yolanda   _____

18. stallions   _____

19. wrestle   _____

20. yawn   _____

STUDY QUESTIONS

1. What is the source of oral cavity obstruction when an oral resonant is produced?

_____

_____

2. What is the phonetic context for intrusion of /j/?

_____

_____

3. What consonant combination represents "q"?

_____

_____

4. What is unique in production of /l/?

_____

_____

5. List five words that contain /r/.

_____

_____

6. Define *approximation*.

_____

_____

CHAPTER

9

Articulation of Vowels

Learning Objectives

After reading this chapter, you will be able to:

1. Define "vowel."

2. State importance of use of Vowel Quadrangle for identifying vowel position.

3. Identify horizontal and vertical tongue reference points used in the Vowel Quadrangle.

4. Explain tongue position for tense and lax vowels.

Vowels play a very special role in our speech by forming the nucleus of a fundamental unit of phonetic structure: the syllable. Syllables were discussed in Chapter 2. Production of vowels differs from consonant production because the tongue does not make contact with a specific articulator for closure. Unlike consonants, vowels are produced with a mostly unobstructed vocal tract. In contrast to consonants, vowels are classified solely by tongue placement to describe *place* of articulation. All vowels are voiced.

Simple vowels are also termed *monophthongs* (defined as *single* sounds). Monophthongs comprise most of the American English vowel system (Lowe & Blosser, 2002).

Diphthongs (defined as *two* sounds) require two articulatory positions as they are produced by rapid gliding from one vowel to another vowel position. Because vowels and diphthongs are required to form a syllable, they are also termed *syllabics*.

Prominent Articulatory Vowel Positions

The vowel quadrangle (Figure 9–1) is a very useful tool to describe vowel production as it provides convenient reference points for specifying tongue position.

171

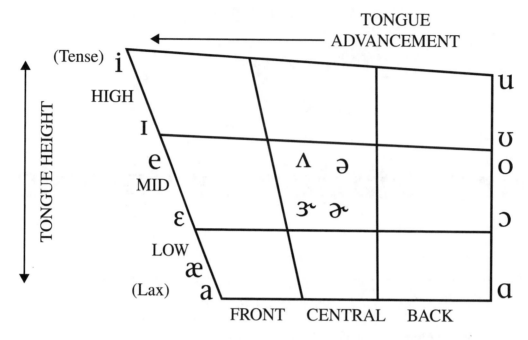

Figure 9–1. The vowel quadrangle.

The position of the *highest point of the arch of the tongue* is considered to be the point of articulation of the vowel. The *vertical dimension* of the vowel quadrangle is known as vowel *height*: high, central (mid), or low. The *horizontal dimension* of the vowel quadrangle, or tongue advancement, identifies how far forward the tongue is located in the oral cavity.

Vowels are also described by the tenseness or laxness of the tongue. A tense vowel requires muscular tension at the root of the tongue. The tongue is elevated and tense for production of the /i/u/e/ vowels. Lax vowels require less muscular tension at the root of the tongue, such as /ɑ/æ/ɚ/. These vowels are produced by a low tongue position in the oral cavity.

After you have studied this chapter and have learned the sound/symbol relationship of vowels, take a movie break and watch *My Fair Lady* (1964). During the movie, you will hear Dr. Peter Ladefoged, who was director of the UCLA Phonetics Laboratory, produce vowel sounds as Dr. Henry Higgins (Rex Harrison) is trying to change Eliza Doolittle's Cockney dialect. Dr. Ladefoged, a pioneer in the field of phonetics, died in 2007.

STUDY QUESTIONS

1. What speech role do vowels play in forming syllables?

   A syllable must contain a vowel or diphthong

2. How does production of vowels differ from consonants?

   Toungue does not make contact with a specific articulator for closure

3. What is the configuration of the vocal tract used for production of vowels?

   The vocal tract is mostly unobstructed.

4. What is difference between monophthongs and diphthongs?

   Monophthong: single sound (one vowel)
   Diphthong: two sounds (two vowels)

5. What does vowel quadrangle provide that is helpful for identifying vowel production?

   Provides reference for tongue

6. What do vertical and horizontal dimensions of the vowel quadrangle indicate for tongue postion?

   Vertical: Height of toungue
   Horizontal: toungue advancement

7. What is the difference between a tense and lax tongue?

   A tense toungue requires muscular tension at roots of toungue; a lax tongue requires less muscular tension at root of toungue.

10

Front Vowels

As the name implies, front vowels of Standard American English are produced in the front of the oral cavity. The tongue is shifted forward to produce /i/ɪ/e/ɛ/æ/. As you say these vowels, you will note that your tongue begins at the highest point in the oral cavity and progresses downward to the lowest point. These vowels are produced with unrounded lips that may be slightly retracted. Some phoneticians include the capped "a" /a/ (used in diphthongs) as a low front vowel.

/i/

Transcription Exercise 10–1

Track: (CD 2, Track 1)

		I	M	F
1.	yes			
2.	leaving		X	
3.	eel	X		
4.	thieves		X	
5.	people		X	
6.	cheapen		X	
7.	quiche		X	
8.	street		X	
9.	helix		X	
10.	hire			

Transcription Exercise 10–2
Vowel: /i/

 Track: (CD 2, Track 2)
Refer to Study Card: 26

Phonetic Symbol	Target Word	Transcription
/i/	1. eat	it
	2. keep	kip
	3. deed	did
	4. key	ki
	5. beak	bik
	6. peak	pik
	7. beet	bit
	8. tea	ti
	9. deep	dip

/i/

Distinctive Features	Tongue Position
High front tense (unrounded) vowel	Tongue moves forward and elevates toward hard palate.
/i/ → (diagram)	Sides of back of tongue close against upper molars.
	Front portion of tongue is raised high in oral cavity.
	Lips are parted slightly.
	Airflow is through the oral cavity.

Voicing/Velopharyngeal Port	Spelling Variations
Voiced—vocal folds *ad*duct.	e *be, me, we*
VP port is closed.	ee *feet, three*
	ea *eat, teach, east*
	ey *key*

Word Positions	Clinical Information
Initial, medial, and final positions in SAE	

/ɪ/

Transcription Exercise 10–3   **Track: (CD 2, Track 3)**

		I	M	F
1.	mild	~~✗~~		
2.	it	✗	~~✗~~	
3.	pixie		✗	
4.	billion		✗	
5.	fine			
6.	guilt		✗	
7.	villain		✗	
8.	sincere		✗	
9.	lymph		✗	
10.	fin		✗	

Transcription Exercise 10–4
Vowel: /ɪ/

 Track: (CD 2, Track 4)
Refer to Study Card: 27

Phonetic Symbol	Target Word	Transcription
/ɪ/	1. kick	kɪk
	2. gig	gɪg
	3. build	bɪld
	4. tick	tɪk
	5. it	ɪt
	6. bit	bɪt
	7. pick	pɪk
	8. kid	kɪd
	9. big	bɪg

/ɪ/

Distinctive Features	Tongue Position
High front lax (unrounded) vowel	Middle to front portion of tongue is raised toward hard palate and alveolar ridge.
	Sides of back of tongue close against upper molars.
	Tip of tongue touches lightly behind lower front teeth.
	Lips are apart.
	Airflow is through the oral cavity.

Voicing/Velopharyngeal Port	Spelling Variations
Voiced—vocal folds *ad*duct.	i *if, in*
VP port is closed.	y *gym, hym*n
	ee b*ee*n
	ui q*ui*z
	o w*o*men
	u b*u*sy

Word Position	Clinical Information
Initial, medial, and final positions in SAE	Referred to as the "short i"
	Many prefer to transcribe using /i/ rather than /ɪ/ in syllables that are unstressed as in "baby" ['bebi]

/ɛ/

Transcription Exercise 10–5

Track: (CD 2, Track 5)

		I	M	F
1.	entail	✗		
2.	penguin		✗	
3.	bell		✗	
4.	mild			
5.	yes		✗	
6.	elf	✗		
7.	gang			
8.	ethic	✗		
9.	guess		✗	
10.	jealous		✗	

Note: The /ɛ/ is frequently substituted with /ɪ/ in Standard American English dialects:

"get" [gɛt] [gɪt]
"pen" [pɛn] [pɪn]

Transcription Exercise 10–6
Vowel: /ɛ/

 Track: (CD 2, Track 6)
Refer to Study Card: 28

Phonetic Symbol	Target Word	Transcription
/ɛ/	1. meld	mɛld
	2. end	ɛnd
	3. dell	dɛl
	4. den	dɛn
	5. led	lɛn
	6. knell	nɛl
	7. dense	dɛnts
	8. sled	slɛd
	9. etch	ɛtʃ

/ε/

Distinctive Features	Tongue Position
Mid-front lax (unrounded) vowel /ε/ ———▶	Sides of back of tongue touch *against* upper molars. Middle to front portion of tongue is raised slightly toward hard palate and alveolar ridge. Tip of tongue touches lightly behind lower front teeth. Lips are apart and neutral. Airflow is through the oral cavity.
Voicing/Velopharyngeal Port	**Spelling Variations**
Voiced—vocal folds *add*uct. VP port is closed.	e *end*, *ebb*, *ten* ea *head*, *steady* ai *said* ie *friend*
Word Positions	**Clinical Information**
Initial and medial positions in SAE	Also known as the epsilon (from the Greek alphabet) or "short e"

/e/

Transcription Exercise 10–7   **Track: (CD 2, Track 7)**

		I	M	F
1.	acorn	✗		
2.	sleigh			✗
3.	vein		✗	
4.	dial			
5.	leisure			
6.	gain		✗	
7.	bag			
8.	lei			✗
9.	attain		✗	
10.	reindeer		✗	

Transcription Exercise 10–8
Vowel: /e/

Track: (CD 2, Track 8)
Refer to Study Card: 29

Phonetic Symbol	Target Word	Transcription
/e/	1. vase	ves
	2. stays	stez
	3. Zane	zen
	4. ate	et
	5. faze	fez
	6. taste	test
	7. face	fes
	8. shave	ʃev
	9. fate	fet

/e/

Distinctive Features	Tongue Position
Mid-front tense (unrounded) vowel	Tongue is raised to mid-portion of oral cavity and shifts forward.
	Tip is at lower front teeth and makes contact with posterior portion of alveolar ridge; tongue contacts upper molars laterally.
/e/	Lips are apart.
	Airflow is through the oral cavity.

Voicing/Velopharyngeal Port	Spelling Variations
Voiced—vocal folds *add*uct.	a *a*che
VP port is closed.	et ball*et*
	ea st*ea*k
	ai g*ai*t
	ee matin*ee*

Word Position	Clinical Information
Initial, medial, and final positions in SAE	Also known as the "long a"
	Some phoneticians use /eɪ/ to represent this sound

/æ/

Transcription Exercise 10–9   Track: (CD 2, Track 9)

		I	M	F
1.	advance	✗	✗	
2.	pan		✗	
3.	ant	✗		
4.	mall			
5.	pain			
6.	dampness		✗	
7.	quack		✗	
8.	cascade		✗	
9.	math		✗	
10.	went			

Transcription Exercise 10–10
Vowel: /æ/

 Track: (CD 2, Track 10)
Refer to Study Card: 30

Phonetic Symbol	Target Word	Transcription
/æ/	1. sash	sæʃ
	2. fast	fæst
	3. ash	æʃ
	4. staff	stæf
	5. vat	væt
	6. shaft	ʃæft
	7. tat	tæt
	8. as	læʃ æz
	9. salve	sæʊ

/æ/

Distinctive Features	Tongue Position
Low front lax (unrounded) vowel /æ/ ⟶	Middle to front portion of tongue is raised toward hard palate, but is low in the mouth so that it rarely contacts upper molars. Tip of tongue is near lower front teeth. Lips are widely separated. Airflow is through the oral cavity. Of all the front vowels, the mandible is in the lowest position.
Voicing/Velopharyngeal Port	**Spelling Variations**
Voiced—vocal folds *ad*duct. VP port is closed.	a *at* ai pl*ai*d ua *g*uarantee au lau*g*h i mer*i*ngue
Word Positions	**Clinical Information**
Initial and medial positions in SAE	Also known as "short a" or "ash"

Crossword Puzzle for /i/, /ɪ/, /ɛ/, /æ/, /e/, and /w/

Answers in Appendix B

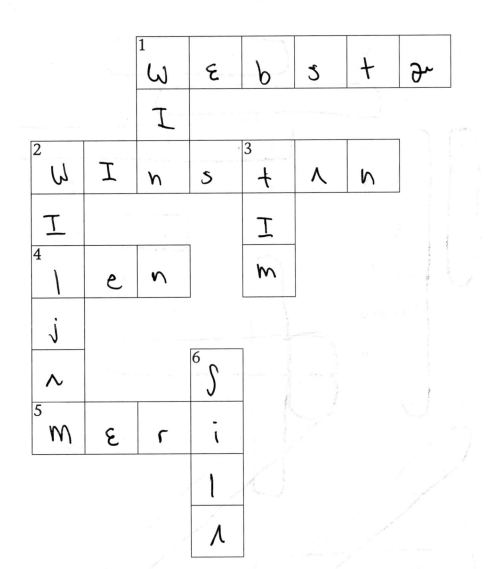

Directions: Transcribe the following words:

Across:
1. Webster
2. Winston
4. Lane
5. Mary

Down:
1. Wynn
2. William
3. Tim
6. Sheila

FOR THE BIRDS

Word Search #13

Answers in Appendix B

```
v   g   e   h   k   g  ·r   i   b   o   w   k
f   ɪ   n   p   i   k   ɑ   k   z   v   m   z
l   i   p   w   ʌ   tʃ ·ɪ   k   ə   d   i   ɔ
o   g   ɛ   ʃ   b   ə   l   d   f   ɛ   v   u
t   ə   r   o   m   s   e   ɛ˞  g   s   g   r
p   l   ə   ɛ   t   f   g   n   d   o   ə   k
i   ð   k   ɚ   l   æ   k   d   v   r   ʃ   i
r   ɝ   i   ʌ   b   l   u   dʒ  e   t   j   w
ɛ   r   t   θ   k   k   dʒ  s   r   m   ɚ   i
n   i   n   n   æ   ə   tʃ  ɪ   t   æ   ɛ   s
ɔ   ŋ   g   m   o   n   n   ə   w   g   ə   f
ʒ   e   r   l   j   h   e   ɛ   ð   p   t   ɪ
h   i   g   r   ɛ   t   z   d   r   aɪ  ŋ   n
m   ɪ   o   l   ɪ   t   v   i   ə   i   i   tʃ
```

Directions: Find and circle the words listed below which contain the front vowels: /i/ɪ/ɛ/æ/e/.

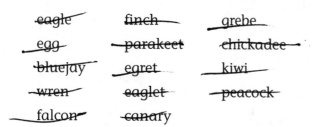

~~eagle~~	~~finch~~	~~grebe~~
~~egg~~	~~parakeet~~	~~chickadee~~
~~bluejay~~	~~egret~~	~~kiwi~~
~~wren~~	~~eaglet~~	~~peacock~~
~~falcon~~	~~canary~~	

Transcription Exercise 10–11
Front Vowels: /i/ɪ/ɛ/e/æ/

Track: (CD 2, Track 11)
Phoneme Study Cards: 26–30

1. flame   flem

2. alley   æli

3. believe   biliv

4. raisin   rezɪn

5. weekday   wikde

6. relax   rilæks

7. ask   æsk

8. people   pipəl

9. remnant   rimnɪnt

10. reign   ~~rirr~~ ren

11. gymnast   dʒɪmnɪst

12. apron   eprɪn

13. namesake   nemsæk

14. busy   bɪzi

15. caffeine   kæfin

16. women   wɪmɪn

17. headache   ~~hed~~ hɛdek

18. please   pliz

19. biscuit   brskɪt

20. eldest   ~~ɛldɛs~~ ɛldɪst

STUDY QUESTIONS

1. What is lip position for front vowels?

   Unrounded slightly reacted

2. /ɪ/ is also referred to as:

   Short "i" "I"

3. What vowel is known as "short a"?

   /æ/

4. List three spelling variations for /ɪ/.

   mid   myth   ~~with~~ built

5. For what front vowel is mandible in lowest position of all front vowels?

   /æ/

6. What front vowel is identified as the "short e"?

   /ɛ/

7. What diphthong do some phoneticians use for /e/?

   /eɪ/

11

Central Vowels

The central vowels are /ə/ʌ/ɚ/ɝ/. As the name indicates, these vowels are produced in the middle (central) portion of the oral cavity, midway between the front and back vowels. The /ə/ and /ɚ/ are classified as unstressed vowels. They are used in unstressed syllables and produced with less force. The /ʌ/ and /ɝ/ used in stressed syllables and produced with more force.

The /ɚ/ and /ɝ/ are also referred to as rhoticized or r-colored vowels due to the influence of the /r/ sound. Garn-Nunn and Lynn (2004) state the /ɝ/ and /r/ differ in these ways: (1) /ɝ/ produced with greater duration, (2) /ɝ/ can form a syllable, (3) tongue moves toward the /r/ consonant production, and (4) unlike /ɝ/, /r/ is voiceless following a voiceless consonant.

This category of vowels usually is difficult for beginning phonetics students to master because it can be difficult to determine whether a stressed or unstressed vowel should be used. Indeed, even seasoned phoneticians may have difficulty transcribing these vowels consistently. Edwards (2003) reports that some phoneticians in America use only the unstressed central vowels (/ə/ɚ/). However, as a student of phonetics, it is important for you to learn use of the central vowels. Transcription Exercises 11–10 through 11–15 provide extra central vowel transcription practice.

/ə/

Transcription Exercise 11–1   **Track: (CD 2, Track 12)**

		I	M	F
1.	ahead	✗		
2.	rattan		✗	
3.	machine		✗	
4.	baton		✗	
5.	cabana			✗
6.	tuba			✗
7.	vanilla			✗
8.	agree	✗		
9.	buffet		✗	
10.	cocoon		✗	

Transcription Exercise 11–2
Vowel: /ə/

 Track: (CD 2, Track 13)
Refer to Study Card: 31

Phonetic Symbol	Target Word	Transcription
/ə/	1. galore	gəˈlor
	2. support	səport
	3. alone	əlon
	4. compose	kəmpos
	5. condone	kəndon
	6. patrol	pətrol
	7. rapport	rəport
	8. ashore	əʃor
	9. lagoon	bəgun

/ə/

Distinctive Features	Tongue Position
Mid-central lax vowel (unrounded, unstressed)	Tongue is flat, but can have a slight arch; tip is at lower front teeth.
	Lips are apart and neutral.
	Airflow is through the oral cavity.

Voicing/Velopharyngeal Port	Spelling Variations
Voiced—vocal folds *ad*duct.	There is no specific letter of the alphabet to represent the schwa. Can substitute for any vowel:
VP port is closed.	a m*a*chine u talc*u*m e r*e*port i hosp*i*tal o pr*o*found ai uncert*ai*n eo pig*eo*n

Word Positions	Clinical Information
Initial, medial, and final positions in SAE	Known as the schwa

Crossword Puzzle for /ə/

Answers in Appendix B

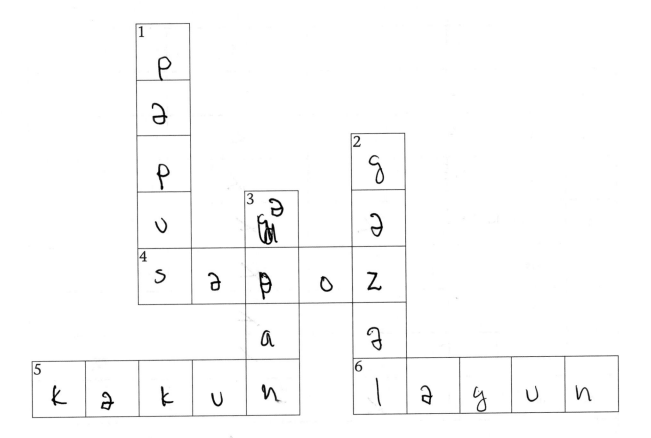

Across:

4. suppose

5. cocoon

6. lagoon

Down:

1. papoose

2. guzzle

3. upon

/ʌ/

Transcription Exercise 11–3   **Track: (CD 2, Track 14)**

		I	M	F
1.	of	✗		
2.	chug		✗	
3.	won		✗	
4.	uncut	✗	✗	
5.	was		✗	
6.	young		✗	
7.	rust		✗	
8.	up	✗		
9.	one		✗	
10.	roost			

Transcription Exercise 11–4
Vowel: /ʌ/

 Track: (CD 2, Track 15)
Refer to Study Card: 32

Phonetic Symbol	Target Word	Transcription
/ʌ/	1. oven	ʌvɪn
	2. touch	tʌtʃ
	3. thumb	θʌm
	4. bum	bʌm
	5. ton	tʌm
	6. pun	pʌn
	7. mutt	mʌt
	8. cud	kʌd
	9. nut	nʌt

/ʌ/

Distinctive Features	Tongue Position
Mid-central vowel (unrounded, stressed)	See tongue position for schwa /ə/
	Tongue may be slightly more retracted as in production for /ɑ/.
	Produced with more muscular tension of the tongue than /ə/.

Voicing/Velopharyngeal Port	Spelling Variations
Voiced—vocal folds *add*uct.	u most frequent and consistent as in p*u*g, s*u*n, h*u*ndred
VP port is closed.	ou r*ou*gh, d*ou*ble
	o t*o*n, s*o*n, t*o*ngue
	oe d*oe*s
	oo bl*oo*d

Word Positions	Clinical Information
Initial and medial positions in SAE	Also referred to as the caret or inverted "v"

Note: The /ʌ/ is used in the popular expression "duh" [dʌ]. Question: Is learning phonetics challenging? Answer: Duh! Or, remember the beginning sounds of the theme to the movie *Jaws*: "duh-duhn . . . "

Crossword Puzzle for /ʌ/

Answers in Appendix B

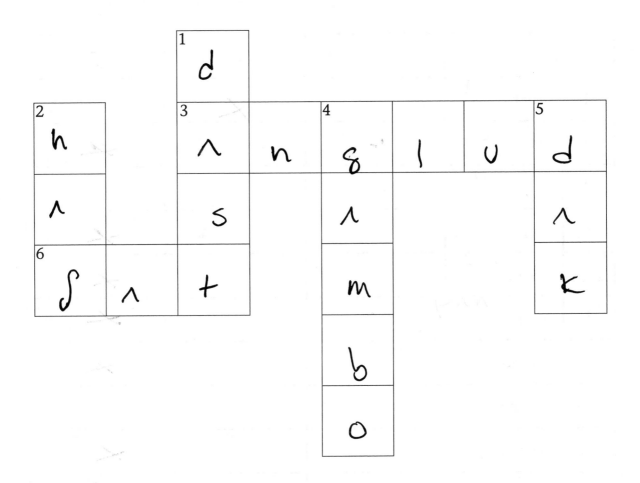

Directions: Transcribe the following words:

Across:
3. unglued
6. shut

Down:
1. dust
2. hush
4. gumbo
5. duck

/ɚ/

Transcription Exercise 11–5   Track: (CD 2, Track 16)

		I	M	F
1.	actor		X	
2.	earner			X
3.	nerd			
4.	sugar			X
5.	anger			X
6.	neighbor			X
7.	creature			X
8.	curtain			
9.	glamour			X
10.	paper			X

Transcription Exercise 11–6
Vowel: /ɚ/

 Track: (CD 2, Track 17)
Refer to Study Card: 33

Phonetic Symbol	Target Word	Transcription
/ɚ/	1. nature	netʃɚ
	2. major	medʒɚ
	3. baker	bekɚ
	4. razor	rezɚ
	5. later	letɚ
	6. pacer	pasɚ
	7. failure	feljɚ
	8. neighbor	nebɚ
	9. safer	sefɚ

/ɚ/

Distinctive Features	Tongue Position
Mid-central r-colored lax vowel (unstressed)	Tongue is slightly elevated from neutral position.
	Sides of tongue close against upper molars.
	Lips are apart.
	Airflow is through the oral cavity.
	Produced with same tongue position as /ɝ/ with the exception that the tongue is more relaxed and duration of this phoneme is shorter than for /ɝ/.

Voicing/Velopharyngeal Port	Spelling Variations
Voiced—vocal folds *ad*duct.	Most often used in unstressed positions of words
VP port is closed.	er butt*er*
	or maj*or*
	our glam*our*
	ur Sat*ur*day
	ure mea*sure*

Word Positions	Clinical Information
Initial, medial, and final positions in SAE	Also known as the hooked schwar or unstressed schwar.

Crossword Puzzle for /ɚ/

Answers in Appendix B

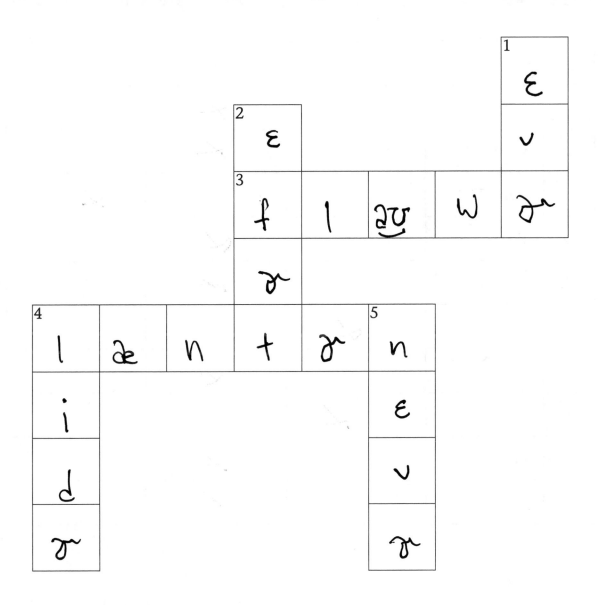

Directions: Transcribe the following words:

Across:

3. flower
4. lantern

Down:

1. ever
2. effort
4. leader
5. never

/ɝ/

Transcription Exercise 11–7   Track: (CD 2, Track 18)

		I	M	F
1.	herb		✗	
2.	worst		✗	
3.	slur			✗
4.	chirp		✓	
5.	surgeon		✗	
6.	urn	✓		
7.	purchase		✗	
8.	earn	✗		
9.	turtle		✗	
10.	myrtle		✗	

Transcription Exercise 11–8
Vowel: /ɝ/

 Track: (CD 2, Track 19)
Refer to Study Card: 34

Phonetic Symbol	Target Word	Transcription
/ɝ/	1. urge	ɝdʒ
	2. verb	vɝb
	3. birth	bɝθ
	4. third	θɝd
	5. dirge	dɝdʒ
	6. burr	bɝ
	7. girth	gɝθ
	8. germ	dʒɝm
	9. earth	ɝθ

i
ɪ   ʌ ə   u ʊ
e   ɝ ɚ   o
ɛ   ɔ
æ   ɑ
a

/ɝ/

Distinctive Features	Tongue Position
Mid-central r-colored tense vowel (stressed) 	Tongue is slightly elevated from neutral position. Sides of tongue close against upper molars. Lips are apart. Airflow is through the oral cavity.

Voicing/Velopharyngeal Port	Spelling Variations
Voiced—vocal folds *ad*duct. VP port is closed.	er h*er*d, m*er*chant, f*er*n ur *ur*ge, f*ur*, t*ur*tle ir ch*ir*p, b*ir*th ear *ear*n, p*ear*l or w*or*m our j*our*ney

Word Positions	Clinical Information
Initial, medial, and final positions in SAE	Also known as the reversed, hooked epsilon and stressed schwar.

Crossword Puzzle for /ɝ/

Answers in Appendix B

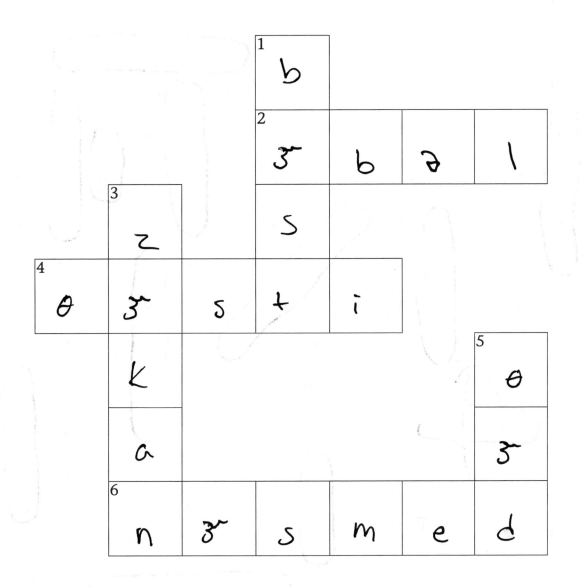

Directions: Transcribe the following words:

Across:
2. herbal
4. thirsty
6. nursemaid

Down:
1. burst
3. zircon
5. third

MID-CENTRAL VOWELS

Word Search #14   Answers in Appendix B

k	p	s	ɝ	θ	k	i	o	s	ɪ	l	v	ɚ	s
r	e	o	z	n	n	p	f	ɛ	l	b	z	ɛ	t
ɛ	ʌ	ð	p	ɛ	d	b	ɝ	t	i	w	ɝ	f	o
k	b	e	h	w	j	r	dʒ	i	d	e	dʒ	ɚ	θ
ɚ	s	h	ɝ	ɑ	p	j	z	θ	ɚ	ʌ	ʊ	t	h
d	b	ʌ	l	h	m	e	u	ɝ	ʍ	ɝ	ɛ	u	dʒ
p	s	f	i	ə	p	m	p	v	n	θ	p	ɝ	ə
n	æ	ɪ	ɚ	n	m	ɛ	d	ɚ	m	ʍ	t	ð	ʌ
d	h	n	o	dʒ	n	ʍ	t	æ	ŋ	e	t	o	h
e	ʃ	ɝ	t	v	g	s	o	n	æ	k	d	ʃ	æ
m	w	s	θ	s	t	p	h	ɑ	g	ɚ	o	g	m
m	j	p	v	t	v	ɝ	ʌ	d	ɚ	z	t	m	ɚ
g	t	i	z	o	t	s	f	n	ɛ	w	tʃ	e	h
t	v	w	ɛ	j	r	w	m	ɑ	d	ɚ	n	dʒ	o

Directions: Find and circle the words listed below which contain the /ɝ/ or /ɚ/ phonemes.

earthquake	nurse	record
urge	modern	effort
earlier	paper	hammer
purse	leader	
shirt	silver	

Transcription Exercise 11–9
Central Vowels: /ə/ʌ/ɚ/ɝ/

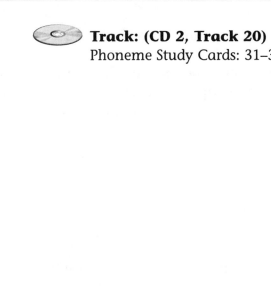

Track: (CD 2, Track 20)
Phoneme Study Cards: 31–34

1. hamburger   hæmbɚgɚ
2. suds   sʌdz
3. kern   kɝn
4. cover   kʌvɚ
5. occur   ʌkɚ
6. fervor   fɝvɚ
7. undone   ʌndʌn
8. eardrum   irdrʌm
9. murmur   mɝmɚ
10. awhile   ɚwaɪl
11. turner   tɝnɚ
12. confirm   kʌnfɝm
13. buzzer   bʌzɚ
14. mature   mʌtʃɚ
15. buffer   tʃɝp
16. chirp   sɝdʒ
17. serge   sɝdʒ
18. verse   vɝs
19. submerge   sʌbmɝdʒ
20. merger   mɝdʒɚ

Transcription Exercise 11–10 **Track: (CD 2, Track 21)**

To help you become familiar with the sound of the schwa /ə/, listen to these words and the transcription. All of these words could be articulated with a different vowel rather than the schwa. For example: "famous" could be transcribed as [femɪs] or [femɛs].

Word	Transcription
1. adore	[əˈdor]
2. often	[ˈaftən]
3. committee	[kəˈmɪti]
4. again	[əˈgɛn]
5. famous	[ˈfeməs]
6. balloon	[bəˈlun]
7. possess	[pəˈzɛs]
8. chagrin	[ʃəˈgrɪn]
9. lapel	[ləˈpɛl]
10. regime	[rəˈʒim]

Transcription Exercise 11–11

Track: (CD 2, Track 22)

Where is the schwa? Listen to these words and decide which vowel has been reduced to the schwa. Remember that the schwa can substitute for any vowel. Answers in Appendix B.

1. cousin _____ cousin _____ kʌzən

2. illness _____ illness _____ Ilnəs

3. distant _____ distant _____ dIstənt

4. promise _____ promise _____ prɑməs

5. palace _____ palace _____ pæləs

6. socket _____ socket _____ sɑkət

7. disease _____ disease _____ dəziz

8. escape _____ escape _____ əskep

9. contain _____ contain _____ kəntən

10. divide _____ divide _____ dəvɑɪd

Transcription Exercise 11–12

Central Vowel Stressed Dictation /ʌ/.

 Track: (CD 2, Track 23)

Listen and transcribe these words. Answers in Appendix B.

1. gulf   gʌlf

2. dust   dʌst

3. dumb   dʌm

4. fuzz   fʌz

5. putt   pʌt

6. plus   plʌs

7. lug   lʌg

8. stuck   stʌk

9. crumb   krʌm

10. plum   plʌm

Transcription Exercise 11–13

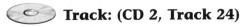 **Track: (CD 2, Track 24)**

Central Vowel Stressed Dictation /ɝ/.

Listen and transcribe these words. Answers in Appendix B.

1. clerk _____klɝk_____

2. first _____fɝst_____

3. heard _____hɝd_____

4. fur _____fɝ_____

5. cursed _____kɝst_____

6. shirk _____ʃɝk_____

7. were _____wɝ_____

8. whirl _____ʊɝl_____

9. per _____pɝ_____

10. curl _____kɝr_____

Transcription Exercise 11–14   **Track: (CD 2, Track 25)**

Listen and transcribe these words which contrast central stressed vowels /ʌ/ and /ɝ/.
Answers in Appendix B.

1. bun   bʌn   burn   bɝn

2. shuck   ʃʌk   shirk   ʃɝk

3. buzz   bʌz   burns   bɝnz

4. hut   hʌt   hurt   hɝt

5. shut   ʃʌt   shirt   ʃɝt

6. cut   kʌt   curt   kɝt

7. luck   lʌk   lurk   lɝk

8. putt   pʌt   pert   pɝt

9. bust   bʌst   burst   bɝst

10. hub   hʌb   Herb   hɝb

Transcription Exercise 11–15   **Track: (CD 2, Track 26)**

Listen and transcribe these words which contain the unstressed central vowel /ɚ/. Answers in Appendix B.

1. plumber   plʌmɚ

2. other   ʌðɚ

3. cluster   klʌstɚ

4. ulcer   ʌlsɚ

5. buffer   bʌfɚ

6. butler   bʌtlɚ

7. plunger   plʌndʒɚ

8. rubber   rʌbɚ

9. southern   sʌðɚn

10. sculpture   skʌlptʃɚ

STUDY QUESTIONS

1. What central vowels are also referred to as rhoticized or r-colored?

/ɚ/   /ɝ/

2. Where in oral cavity are central vowels produced?

Middle of the oral cavity

3. List four ways /ɝ/ and r differ.

/ɝ/ produced with greater duration / tongue moves towards the /r/ constant

/ɝ/ can form a syllable / /r/ is voiceless following a voiceless constant

4. The schwa is also referred to as:

The middle mid-central lax vowel

5. What popular expression is /ʌ/ used in?

"Ouh."

6. What central vowel is also referred to as hooked schwar or unstressed schwar?

/ɚ/

7. Is /ʌ/ used in stressed or unstressed syllables?

Stressed

12

Back Vowels

Learning Objectives

After reading this chapter, you will be able to:

1. State tongue position for all back vowels and how they are produced.

2. Identify lip position for back vowels.

3. List spelling variations for back vowels.

4. Transcribe words using back vowels.

As the name indicates, the back vowels /u/ʊ/o/ɔ/ɑ/ are produced in the back portion of the oral cavity. The posterior portion of the tongue is elevated toward the velum. The tongue tip is behind the lower central incisors or may lightly touch the lower alveolar ridge. The /ɑ/ has the greatest mandibular opening of all American English vowel sounds (Garn-Nunn & Lynn, 2004). With the exception of /ɑ/, the lips round or slightly protrude for production of the back vowels.

/u/

Transcription Exercise 12–1   Track: (CD 2, Track 27)

		I	M	F
1.	noodle		✗	
2.	do			✗
3.	dew			✗
4.	should			
5.	ooze	✗		
6.	suit		✗	
7.	boutique		✗	
8.	fool		✗	
9.	duke		✗	
10.	two			✗

Transcription Exercise 12–2
Vowel: /u/

 Track: (CD 2, Track 28)
Refer to Study Card: 35

Phonetic Symbol	Target Word	Transcription
/u/	1. rule	rʊl
	2. sue	sʊ
	3. loose	ⱷ lʊs
	4. rue	rʊ
	5. loop	lʊp
	6. flew	flʊ
	7. sloop	ʃlʊp
	8. pool	pʊl
	9. fool	fʊl

/u/

Distinctive Features	Tongue Position
High back tense rounded vowel 	Back of tongue is raised high and tense in oral cavity. Sides of back of tongue close against upper molars. Tongue tip is behind lower front teeth. Lips are rounded.

Voicing/Velopharyngeal Port	Spelling Variations
Voiced—vocal folds *ad*duct. VP port is closed.	Occurs most frequently as "oo" as in b*oo*t, c*oo*l, t*oo* o d*o*, wh*o* ew bl*ew*, gr*ew* ou s*ou*p, gr*ou*p ui fr*ui*t, br*ui*se R*oo*f, r*oo*t, h*oo*p can be pronounced with either /u/ or /ʊ/

Word Position	Clinical Information
Medial and final position in SAE	Rarely occurs in Initial position in SAE, such as "*oops*"

/ʊ/

Transcription Exercise 12–3   **Track: (CD 2, Track 29)**

		I	M	F
1.	full		✗	
2.	oops	✗	✗	
3.	wolf		✗	
4.	mutt		✗	
5.	soot		✗	
6.	goof		✗	
7.	whoops		✗	
8.	sugar		✗	
9.	footstool		✗	
10.	hood		✗	

Transcription Exercise 12–4
Vowel: /ʊ/

 Track: (CD 2, Track 30)
Refer to Study Card: 36

Phonetic Symbol	Target Word	Transcription
/ʊ/	1. cook	kʊ
	2. wool	wʊl
	3. foot	fʊt
	4. wood	wʊd
	5. look	~~fo~~ lʊk
	6. wolf	wʊlf
	7. full	fʊl
	8. could	cʊd
	9. nook	nʊk

/ʊ/

Distinctive Features	Tongue Position
High back lax rounded vowel 	Sides of back of tongue close lightly against upper molars. Sides of back of tongue close lightly against upper molars. Back of tongue is raised high in oral cavity. Tongue tip touches behind lower front teeth. Teeth are slightly open. Lips are rounded. Airflow is through the oral cavity.
Voicing/Velopharyngeal Port	**Spelling Variations**
Voiced—vocal folds *ad*duct. VP port is closed.	oo *book, look, wool* u p*u*ll ou c*ou*ld, w*ou*ld
Word Position	**Clinical Information**
Medial position only in SAE	Also known as the upsilon or capped "u"

/o/

Transcription Exercise 12–5   **Track: (CD 2, Track 31)**

		I	M	F
1.	old	✗		
2.	moot			
3.	sew			✗
4.	lotion		✗	
5.	mow			✗
6.	who			
7.	cola		✗	
8.	toast		✗	
9.	bowl		✗	
10.	macho			✗

Transcription Exercise 12–6
Vowel: /o/

 Track: (CD 2, Track 32)
Refer to Study Card: 37

Phonetic Symbol	Target Word	Transcription
/o/	1. note	not
	2. tone	ton
	3. own	on
	4. tote	tot
	5. know	no
	6. oat	ot
	7. hone	hon
	8. no	no
	9. owe	o

/o/

Distinctive Features	Tongue Position
Mid-back tense rounded vowel	Body of tongue shifts slightly back of center and is raised.
	Tongue tip contacts lower front teeth.
	Lips round and protrude.

/O/

Voicing/Velopharyngeal Port	Spelling Variations
Voiced—vocal folds *ad*duct.	o *old, go, no*
VP port is closed.	oa c*oa*t, b*oa*t
	ow cr*ow*, kn*ow*
	oe d*oe*
	ew s*ew*

Word Positions	Clinical Information
Initial, medial, and final position in SAE	Some phoneticians refer to this phoneme as the diphthong /oʊ/

/ɔ/

Transcription Exercise 12–7   **Track: (CD 2, Track 33)**

		I	M	F
1.	all	✗		
2.	thong		✗	
3.	sauce		✗	
4.	awe	✗		
5.	schwa			✗
6.	moth		✗	
7.	pa			✗
8.	squaw			✗
9.	paw			✗
10.	thought		✗	

Note: Dependent on geographic location, speakers may use /a/ when pronouncing these words.

Transcription Exercise 12–8
Vowel: /ɔ/

 Track: (CD 2, Track 34)
Refer to Study Card: 38

Phonetic Symbol	Target Word	Transcription
/ɔ/	1. sought	sɔt
	2. bawdy	bɔdi
	3. wrought	wrɔt
	4. prawn	prɔn
	5. call	kɔl
	6. taut	tɔt
	7. thought	θɔt
	8. vault	vɔlt
	9. lawful	lɔfʊl

Note: Dependent on geographic location, speakers may use /a/ when pronouncing these words.

/ɔ/

Distinctive Features	Tongue Position
Low Mid-back lax rounded vowel	Back and middle portion of tongue slightly raised.
	Tongue tip touches behind lower front incisors.
	Lips round and protrude slightly.

Voicing/Velopharyngeal Port	Spelling Variations
Voiced—vocal folds *adduct*.	au *auto, applause, laundry*
VP port is closed.	aw *awe, lawn, jaw*
	augh(t) *caught, taught*
	o *off, strong*
	a *ball, call*

Word Positions	Clinical Information
Initial, medial, and final position in SAE	Also referred to as the "open o" or "reversed c"
	Edwards (2003) finds this sound very interesting. The /ɔ/ can be affected by a speaker's dialiect. The /ɔ/ is not used consistently in Standard American English.

/a/

Transcription Exercise 12–9

Track: (CD 2, Track 35)

		I	M	F
1.	pasta		✗	
2.	almond	✗		
3.	spa			✗
4.	launch		✗	
5.	genre		✗	
6.	yacht		✗	
7.	aqua	✗		
8.	lunch			
9.	schwa			✗
10.	entree	✗		

Transcription Exercise 12–10
Vowel: /ɑ/

 Track: (CD 2, Track 36)
Refer to Study Card: 39

Phonetic Symbol	Target Word	Transcription
/ɑ/	1. ah	ɑ
	2. not	nɑt
	3. ha	hɑ
	4. yacht	jɑt
	5. tot	tɑt
	6. yon	jɑn
	7. haunt	hɑnt
	8. taught	tɑt
	9. aunt	ɑnt

Note: Dependent on geographic location, speakers may use /ɔ/ when pronouncing these words.

/ɑ/

Distinctive Features	Tongue Position
Low back lax unrounded vowel	Tongue is slightly raised in back.
	Tip touches behind lower front teeth.
	Lips do not round or protrude.

← /ɑ/

Voicing/Velopharyngeal Port	Spelling Variations
Voiced—vocal folds *ad*duct.	o p*o*t, d*o*t, *o*live
VP port is closed.	a he*a*rt
	en *e*ncore

Word Positions	Clinical Information
Initial, medial, and final position in SAE	Used to transcribe the popular expression "ah"

Crossword Puzzle for /u/, /ʊ/, /o/, /ɑ/, and /ɔ/

Answers in Appendix B

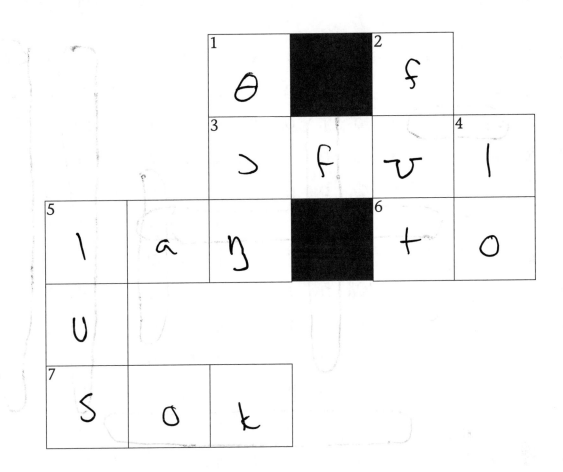

Directions: Transcribe the following words:

Across:
3. awful
5. long
6. toe
7. soak

Down:
1. thong
2. foot
4. low
5. loose

BACK VOWELS

Word Search #15

Answers in Appendix B

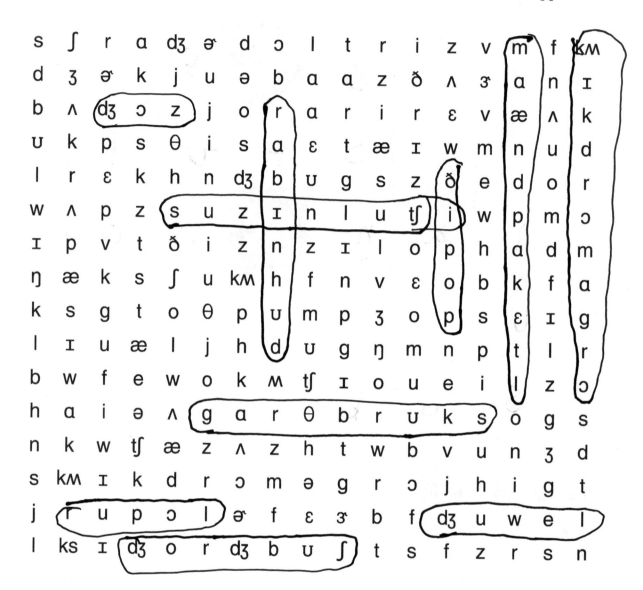

Directions: Find and circle the words which contain the /u/ʊ/o/ɑ/ɔ/ phonemes.

The Popa	Jewel
Garth Brooks	RuPaul
Ma and Pa Kettle	Robin Hood
George Bush	Quick Draw McGraw
Jaws	Susan Lucci

Transcription Exercise 12–11
Back Vowels: /u/ʊ/o/ɔ/a/

 Track: (CD 2, Track 37)
Phoneme Study Cards: 35–39

1. coupon   kupɑn
2. hook   hʊk
3. encore   ankor
4. hawthorn   haθɔrn
5. newsroom   nuzrum
6. taco   tako
7. yoyo   jojo
8. awful   ɔfʊl
9. yacht   jat
10. lollipop   lalipap
11. cookbook   cʊkbʊk
12. boastful   bostfʊl
13. footstool   fʊtstʊl
14. horseshoe   ~~horsf~~ horsʃu
15. fought   ~~fɑt~~ fɔt
16. dorm room   dorm rum
17. fruit   frut
18. mothball   maθbɔl
19. soak   sok
20. thoughtful   θɔtfʊl

STUDY QUESTIONS

1. Which back vowel has greatest mandibular opening?

   /ɑ/

2. What is the lip position for the majority of back vowels?

   Lips round or slightly protrude

3. What is the Greek name for /ʊ/?

   Upsilon

4. Which back vowels are produced with rounded lips?

   /ʊ/ u/ o

5. List four words that contain the /ʊ/ phoneme.

   bushel   crook   woules   put

CHAPTER

13

Diphthongs

Learning Objectives

After reading this chapter, you will be able to:

1. Define diphthong.

2. Explain how a diphthong is produced.

3. State what is used to indicate how two vowels sounds are used together.

4. Identify which diphthongs are offglides and onglides.

5. Transcribe words using diphthongs.

A *diphthong* represents two vowels that are spoken one after the other in continuation, as in saying a single vowel. The first vowel rapidly "glides" into the position of the second vowel. Simply, a diphthong begins by approximating the articulatory position of one vowel and ends by approximating the articulatory position of another vowel. It should be noted that *diphthong* can be pronounced in two ways: [dɪfθɑŋ] or [dɪpθɑŋ].

Diphthongs are not just the sum total of one vowel plus another but are a grad-ual movement of the articulators from one position to another. Figure 13–1 illustrates this movement. You will notice that the "capped a" is a component of the /aɪ/ and /aʊ/ diphthongs.

To indicate that the two vowel sounds in each diphthong are used together, a slur ‿ is used. The diphthongs /aɪ/ /aʊ/ and /ɔɪ/ are off-glides, made with the tongue moving from a lower vowel to a high vowel position. The /ju/ is an on-glide, with movement from a higher sound to a lower vowel position.

DIPHTHONGS

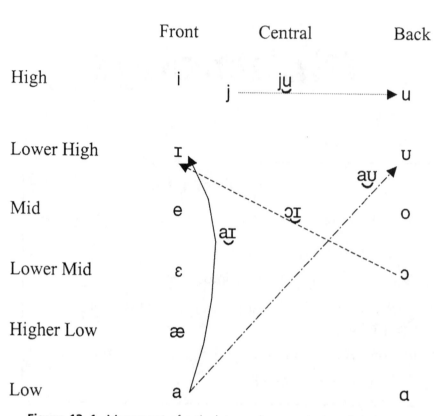

Figure 13–1. Movement of articulators when producing diphthongs.

/aɪ/

Transcription Exercise 13–1

Track: (CD 2, Track 38)

		I	M	F
1.	island	✕		
2.	eye	✕		
3.	guy			✕
4.	minus		✕	
5.	dial		✕	
6.	rhyme		✕	
7.	sweet			
8.	high			✕
9.	niece			
10.	bride		✕	

Transcription Exercise 13–2
Diphthong: /aɪ/

 Track: (CD 2, Track 39)
Refer to Study Card: 40

Phonetic Symbol	Target Word	Transcription
/aɪ/	1. buy	baɪ
	2. cider	saɪdɚ
	3. height	haɪt
	4. feisty	faɪsti
	5. slice	slaɪs
	6. thyme	taɪm
	7. write	raɪt
	8. sigh	saɪ
	9. rhyme	raɪm

/aɪ/

Distinctive Features	Tongue Position
Rising low front to high front (off-glide) diphthong	Tongue is low in the oral cavity. Tongue moves from low front position of /a/ to high front position of /ɪ/.
Voicing/Velopharyngeal Port	**Spelling Variations**
Voiced—vocal folds *ad*duct. VP port is closed.	i w*i*ld, ch*i*ld, *i*dea ia d*i*amond i-e b*i*ke, *i*ce, k*i*te y fr*y*, m*y*, wh*y* ie cr*i*ed, p*i*e, l*i*e igh he*igh*t, n*igh*
Word Positions	**Clinical Information**
Initial, medial, and final positions in SAE	Also referred to as the "long i"

/aʊ/

Transcription Exercise 13–3   Track: (CD 2, Track 40)

		I	M	F
1.	ouch	✗		
2.	lawn			
3.	coward		✗	
4.	vowel		✗	
5.	how			✗
6.	toffee			
7.	shout		✗	
8.	know			
9.	lounge		✗	
10.	house		✗	

Transcription Exercise 13–4
Diphthong: /aʊ/

 Track: (CD 2, Track 41)
Refer to Study Card: 41

Phonetic Symbol	Target Word	Transcription
/aʊ/	1. oust	aʊst
	2. trout	traʊt
	3. gouging	gaʊʤɪdʒɪŋ
	4. prowl	praʊwəl
	5. chowder	tʃaʊdɚ
	6. household	haʊshold
	7. bound	baʊnd
	8. louse	laʊs
	9. bough	baʊ

/aʊ/

Distinctive Features	Tongue Position
Rising low front to high back (off-glide) diphthong	Tongue is in low front position for /a/ and glides back to high back position of /ʊ/.

/U/ →

/a/ →

Voicing/Velopharyngeal Port	Spelling Variations
Voiced—vocal folds *add*uct. VP port is closed.	ou *out*, *house*, th*ou* ow *owl*, *town*, v*ow*

Word Positions	Clinical Information
Initial, medial, and final positions in SAE	

/ɔɪ/

Transcription Exercise 13–5   Track: (CD 2, Track 42)

		I	M	F
1.	coy			✗
2.	choice		✗	
3.	town			
4.	join		✗	
5.	cipher			
6.	moist		✗	
7.	mist			
8.	buoyant		✗	
9.	juice			
10.	spoil		✗	

Transcription Exercise 13–6
Diphthong: /ɔɪ/

 Track: (CD 2, Track 43)
Refer to Study Card: 42

Phonetic Symbol	Target Word	Transcription
/ɔɪ/	1. hoisting	hɔɪstɪŋ
	2. coiled	kɔɪld
	3. destroy	dɛstrɔɪ
	4. foils	fɔɪlz
	5. loiter	lɔɪtɚ
	6. voicing	vɔɪsɪŋ
	7. toy	tɔɪ
	8. exploit	ɛksplɔɪt
	9. avoid	əvɔɪd

/ɔɪ/

Distinctive Features	Tongue Position
Rising mid-back to high front (off-glide) diphthong	Tongue glides from lower mid-back position of /ɔ/ to high front /ɪ/; lips unround.

/ɪ/

/ɔ/

Voicing/Velopharyngeal Port	Spelling Variations
Voiced—vocal folds *ad*duct. VP port is closed.	oi *oi*l, c*oi*n oy *oy*ster, l*oy*al, j*oy*

Word Position	Clinical Information
Initial, medial, and final positions in SAE	Also transcribed as /ɔ̞ɪ/

/ju/

Transcription Exercise 13–7   Track: (CD 2, Track 44)

		I	M	F
1.	few			✗
2.	union	✗		
3.	beauty		✗	
4.	cute		✗	
5.	pew			✗
6.	use	✗		
7.	huge		✗	
8.	fool			
9.	humor		✗	
10.	hula			

Transcription Exercise 13–8
Diphthong: /ju/

 Track: (CD 2, Track 45)
Refer to Study Card: 43

Phonetic Symbol	Target Word	Transcription
/ju/	1. uke	juk
	2. fuchsia	fjuʃə
	3. music	mjuzɪk
	4. huge	hjudʒ
	5. mutant	mjutɪnt
	6. pupil	pjupəl
	7. spewed	spjud
	8. butte	bjut
	9. fume	fjum

/ju/

Distinctive Features	Tongue Position
High front to high back on-glide diphthong	Tip is at lower front teeth.
	Body of tongue is raised toward hard palate.
	Tongue moves to high back position of /u/.

Voicing/Velopharyngeal Port	Spelling Variations
Voiced—vocal folds *add*uct.	u *u*nit
VP port is closed.	u-e *use*
	eau b*eau*ty
	ew f*ew*

Word Positions	Clinical Information
Initial, medial, and final positions in SAE	

Crossword Puzzle for /aɪ/, /aʊ/, /ɔɪ/, and /ju/

Answers in Appendix B

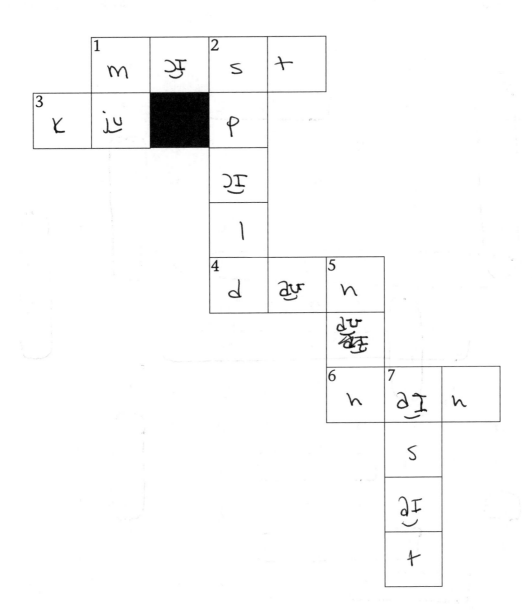

Directions: Transcribe the following words:

Across:

1. moist
3. cue
4. down
6. nine

Down:

1. mew
2. spoiled
5. noun
7. eyesight

DIPHTHONGS

Word Search #16

Answers in Appendix B

```
s   ʃ   r   d   o   n   p   ɚ   r   c   t   t   v
h   aɪ  æ   k   s   v   ju  z   p   n   ə   v   ʌ
d   s   t   ə   ɛ   c   ɛ   b   c   ɔɪ  n   r   d
b   h   i   n   b   w   w   r   b   s   z   f   k
s   aʊ  ɛ   t   k   z   ʌ   u   ʊ   t   i   h   p
h   s   aʊ  θ   b   aʊ  n   d   m   ɚ   b   ju  s
f   p   ʒ   m   ɪ   g   z   i   m   ʒ   u   m   n
k   æ   w   aɪ  l   d   f   aʊ  l   æ   ʊ   ɚ   p
l   ɛ   t   n   æ   k   h   ʌ   ɪ   k   s   n   æ
b   b   s   θ   p   ə   r   z   d   p   i   g   s
h   ɪ   f   ŋ   s   ɔɪ  l   v   z   ɔɪ  v   ʒ   z
n   ju  æ   l   ks  dʒ  t   ʃ   e   z   i   z   f
s   b   z   f   ju  ʃ   ə   t   r   w   g   c   aɪ
o   ɪ   k   aʊ  tʃ  g   j   r   æ   m   ɑ   ɚ   j
```

Directions: Find and circle the words listed below which contain the /aɪ/aʊ/ɔɪ/ju/ phonemes.

icehouse	wildfowl	soil
fuchsia	high	mine
poise	humor	oyster
you	views	couch
southbound		

Transcription Exercise 13–9
Diphthongs: /aɪ/aʊ/ɔɪ/ju/

 Track: (CD 2, Track 46)
Phoneme Study Cards: 40–43

1. foundry   faʊndri

2. join   dʒɔɪn

3. Yukon   juˈkɑn

4. brine   braɪn

5. toil   tɔɪl

6. January   dʒænjuwɛri

7. oust   aʊst

8. ukulele   jukəleli

9. moist   mɔɪst

10. amulet   æmjulɛt

11. pout   paʊt

12. byte   baɪt

13. noun   ~~naʊn~~ naʊn

14. noise   nɔɪz

15. frowning   fraʊnɪŋ

16. I   aɪ

17. contributor   kʌntrɪbjutɚ

18. oink   ɔɪŋk

19. mime   maɪm

20. brownies   braʊniz

STUDY QUESTIONS

1. What does a diphthong represent?

   Two vowels spoken in sequence

2. Why are diphthongs not considered a combination of vowels?

   Gradual movement of the articulators from one vowel to another

3. How is slur written?

   To Indicate two vowel sounds in each dipthong are used together

4. What diphthongs are off-glides?

   /aɪ/   /aʊ/   /ɔɪ/

5. What is the onglide diphthong?

   /ju/

6. What diphthong is referred to as "long i"?

   /aɪ/

CHAPTER

14

Word Stress

Learning Objectives

After reading this chapter, you will be able to:

1. Define stress as it relates to syllables.

2. Identify three features associated with stress.

3. Describe how stress can change a noun to a verb.

4. State four ways to determine syllable stress.

5. Explain use of stress and morphological markers.

6. Identify primary stress in two to four syllable words.

This chapter reviews the basics of stress. The term *stress* is often used interchangeably with the term *accent*. Stress refers to the most prominent part of a syllable in a multisyllabic word or word within a phrase. Greater breath force creates this emphasis. Singh (2006) states stress has been associated with (a) high amplitude (loudness), (b) long duration of the syllable nucleus (time), and (c) high frequency (pitch) of the syllable nucleus. Singh concludes that stressing syllables or words requires increased effort on the part of the speaker. He also adds that the result is that some words or parts of words stand out more than others, making it easier for the listener to grasp the most important meaningful elements of the message.

In words of more than one syllable, one syllable will usually receive more stress than the other. For example, the first syllable of "hap-py" receives more stress than the second syllable. In addition, stress can serve a *phonemic* function. A change in stressed syllable changes word meaning. For example, the first syllable of the noun "'rebel" receives primary (or greatest) stress. However, if the second syllable is stressed, it is changed into the verb re'bel.

Determining stress is not always easy. Garn-Nunn and Lynn (2004) view assignment of stress in English as very erratic due to the speaker following conventional usage. American English speakers are familiar with word pronunciation. This is an area where English second-language learners can have difficulty. One *very simple* way in which to determine syllable stress is to place stress on the *wrong* syllable. If you heard someone say "IMportant" rather than "imPORtant" it would sound unusual to you. Figure 14–1 provides an example of how stress in a word can produce a laugh.

Here are some helpful hints to determine stress:

1 One-syllable words spoken in isolation always receive primary stress.

2 The majority of two-syllable words have stress on the first syllable.

3 Compound verbs have primary stress on the second verb, such as in "over*throw*."

4 Compound words of two syllables have the same amount of stress on each word (cupcake).

The International Phonetic Association alphabet suggests using three distinct stress levels in English multisyllabic words described as: (a) *primary stress* with the stress mark ['] in front of the syllable receiving primary stress, (b) *secondary stress* [ˌ], (c) and no symbol to indicate *unstress*. However, the "stress" of this chapter focuses on assigning primary stress on the first or second syllable as this can be most helpful. The

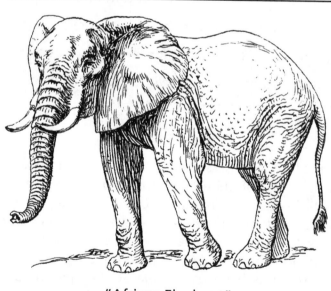

"African Elephant"
(Af-rican)

Figure 14–1. An example of how changing the stress of a word can make an amusing difference: *From the journal of a preschool teacher:* All of my five-year-old students are learning to read. Yesterday, one student pointed to a picture in a zoo book and said, "Look! It's a frickin' elephant!" I took a deep breath, then asked, "What did you call it?" The child responded, "It's a frickin' elephant! It says so on the picture!" And so it did . . .

reader is referred to Edwards (2003) and Singh (2006) for further discussion of secondary stress.

Adding a prefix or suffix usually does not cause a change in primary stress. Table 14–1 provides examples of morphological markers.

Table 14–1. Syllable Stress and Examples of Morphological Markers

Morphological Marker	Base Word	Number of Syllables	Primary Syllable Stress		Transcription
			1st	2nd	
Regular plural -s	plants	1	X		[plænts]
Regular plural -z	signs	1	X		[saɪnz]
Regular plural -ez	bunches	2	X		[bʌntʃɛz]
3rd Person					
Regular plural -s	sits	1	X		[sɪts]
Regular plural -z	runs	1	X		[rʌnz]
Regular plural -ez	crashes	2	X		[kræʃɛz]
Regular past tense -t	walked	1	X		[wakt]
Regular past tense -d	plugged	1	X		[plʌgd]
Regular past tense -ed	waited	2	X		[wetɪd]
Present progressive -ing	walking	2	X		[wɔlkɪŋ]

Important Note: As you can see, prefixes and suffixes (including possessives and modifiers) do not have primary stress on the second syllable.

Exercise 14–1   **Track: (CD 2, Track 47)**

This exercise provides practice in identifying primary stress in two syllable words. Listen carefully to hear which syllable is stressed. Stressed syllable is in **bold** print.

First Syllable Primary Stress↗	Second Syllable Primary Stress↗
1. **teach**er	1. de**ter**
2. **prior**	2. a**bove**
3. **mor**al	3. o**bey**
4. **sadd**le	4. sham**poo**
5. **happy**	5. a**mass**
6. **taco**	6. in**fect**
7. **fad**ed	7. be**side**
8. **injure**	8. re**main**
9. **careful**	9. a**fraid**
10. **funny**	10. as**sist**

Transcription Exercise 14–2   Track: (CD 2, Track 48)

Listen to these words in which primary stress changes the meaning of the word. The first five have been completed for you. See Appendix B for answers.

1. 'digest   1. di' gest

2. 'contest   2. con' test

3. 'rebel   3. re' bel

4. 'produce   4. pro' duce

5. 'address   5. ad' dress

6. __'record__   6. __'re cord__

7. __'in valid__   7. __in 'valid__

8. __'desert__   8. __de 'sert__

9. __'refuse__   9. __re 'fuse__

10. __'present__   10. __pre 'sent__

Transcription Exercise 14–3 **Track: (CD 2, Track 49)**

After listening to these words pronounced on the CD, decide which syllable has primary stress in these two, three and four syllable words. Remember to place the primary stress mark before the syllable which has primary stress. Answers in Appendix B.

		Syllable Division	# of Syllables
1.	licorice	lic ‑or ‑ice	3
2.	ingredient	in · gre · di · ent	4
3.	crying	cry · ing	2
4.	another	a · no th · er	3
5.	audible	aud · di · ble	3
6.	hilarious	hi · lar · i · ous	4
7.	security	se · cu · ri · ty	4
8.	computer	com · pu · ter	3
9.	saxophone	sax · o · phone	3
10.	bigger	big · ger	2
11.	pleasure	plea · sure	2
12.	aggravation	ag · gra · va · tion	4
13.	aftermath	af · ter · math	3
14.	resource	re · source	2
15.	prepare	pre · pare	2
16.	liberal	lib · er · al	3
17.	watermelon	wa · ter · mel · on	4
18.	generation	gen · er · a · tion	4
19.	evaporate	e · vap · o · rate	4
20.	public	pub · lic	2

STUDY QUESTIONS

1. What is another term for stress?

Accent

2. Define stress.

Most prominent part of a syllable in a multisyllabic word or word in a phrase

3. How does stress function to change noun to verb?

Stress Placed on 1st or 2nd syllable.

4. How do morphological markers affect word stress?

Majority of morphological markers do not change stress in a word. The stress is usually on the root word & first syllable of a two-syllable word

5. How are components of compound words of two syllables stressed?

Words of two syllables have the same amount of stress

6. According to Singh, name three features of stress.

Stress has been associated with : (a) high amplitude (loudness), (b) long duration of the syllable nucleus (time), and (c) high frequency (pitch) of the syllable nucleus.

15

Dynamics of Connected Speech

Learning Objectives

After reading this chapter, you will be able to:

1. Define accommodation and state two types.

2. State difference between progressive and regressive assimilation.

3. Describe process of intrusion of /t/ in the word "mince."

4. Define diacritic and give examples in words.

5. Explain co-articulation.

6. Define phonetic environment/context.

Introduction

By the time you read this chapter, you have spent numerous hours studying the IPA to memorize the phonetic symbols and completing the Transcription Exercises. In this chapter, you will learn about the interesting changes in words that can occur during speech. The renowned linguist, Peter Ladefoged, compares the rapid tongue move- ments required for speech to that of a concert pianist's rapid finger movements (2005, p. 185). During speech, considerable effort is expended by muscles of the tongue, jaw, lips, velum, and laryngeal region to produce the finely timed precision move- ments required to distinctly articulate each phoneme. According to Shipley and McAfee (2008), conversational speech is uttered at the incredible speed of 270 words per minute.

To cope with this task of articulating extremely rapid changes from phoneme to phoneme, *accommodation* occurs. Accommodation is an adjustment or adaptation of a speech sound as a result of the *phonetic environment* (or *context*) of a phoneme. Phonetic environment describes the phonemes that surround a specific speech sound. There are two types of accommodation, *assimilation* and *coarticulation.*

Assimilation produces major changes that occur when a phoneme is omitted, added, or changed to a different phoneme.

Coarticulation produces minor changes in phonemes. Phoneticians disagree on whether the processes of coarticulation and assimilation are two distinct processes or are similar. We support MacKay (1987) in his view of two processes.

Assimilation

There are two types of assimilation: *progressive* and *regressive assimilation.* These types of assimilation can result in a change in place of production and/or voicing of a phoneme.

Progressive Assimilation

Say the word "dogs." When articulated, the word is transcribed as [dɑgz]. Progressive assimilation has occurred in this word in a left to right pattern. The voicing of the /g/ has influenced the unvoiced /s/, changing it into the voiced /z/. The *preceding* phoneme /g/ has influenced the phoneme which follows, /s/. Progressive assimilation occurs as a function of *morphology,* or the study of *morphemes.* According to McLaughlin (2006), a *morpheme* is a minimal, meaningful unit of language. Of the two types of morphemes, free and bound, we focus on the *bound* morphemes, which must be attached to a word.

Some examples of these are the -s [kɑfs] and -z forms [sʌnz] and the past tense -t [rekt]. Transcription Exercise 15–1 will give you practice for this concept.

Another example of progressive assimilation occurs in the word "horseshoe." The final sound of /s/ in "horse" is completely assimilated into the prolonged initial sound of "shoe" /ʃ/, so the word is transcribed as [horʃu].

Regressive Assimilation

In contrast to progressive assimilation, the effects of regressive assimilation occur in a right to left manner. In this type of assimilation, a phoneme is changed by the phoneme that *follows* it. For example, in the word "bank," the /k/ influences the preceding /n/ phoneme by changing it into an /ŋ/. The correct transcription would be [beŋk].

Unless each phoneme is produced with a pause before and after as in "b-a-n-k" (which would sound unusual), the effects of regressive assimilation cannot be avoided. The reason this occurs is that the place of articulation of the /k/ (lingua-velar) affects the place of articulation of the /n/ (lingua-alveolar), and the /n/ *assimilates* the place of articulation of the /ŋ/, which is also a lingua-velar.

Transcription Exercise 15–1 contains opportunities for transcription of words with regressive assimilation.

Phonemes can also be omitted during speech. The word "veteran" [vɛtɚɪn] is often pronounced [vɛtrɪn]. Omission, also called *elision,* occurs very frequently in phrases. The phrase, "Where have you been?" can be shortened to [wɛrjʌbɪn].

In contrast to phoneme elimination, some sounds can be added, a process known as *epenthesis* or *intrusion.* The /t/ phoneme is a common intrusive sound, especially when a nasal sound is followed by an unvoiced sound. Say the word "mince." An interesting thing occurs when the word "mince" is articulated. Unless we pause between saying the /n/ and /s/ sounds (which would sound unusual), the word is articulated as [mɪnᵗs]. You will notice the addition of the /t/ which has been intruded. In producing the word "mince," the tongue is at the alveolar ridge for the /n/, which is also where the /s/ is produced. To make articulation easier, the tongue *remains* at the alveolar ridge, with the result of the intruded /t/. The /n,s,t/ are all produced in the same *place* of articulation. Intrusion is defined as the addition of a sound which is not included in the spelling of the word but which occurs when the word is articulated.

Remember that the intruded sound may or not be audible, but is present because it is articulated. Some phoneticians choose to raise the intruded /t/ when a word is transcribed. Intrusion is a result of the speed with which we speak and economical articulatory movements.

The /p/ and /k/ phonemes are also subject to intrusion. The word "warmth" is transcribed as [wormpθ] with the intrusion of the /p/. In order to eliminate the intruded /p/, the speaker would have to pause between saying the /m/ and the /θ/. An example of the intruded /k/ occurs in the word "length," which is articulated as [leŋkθ]. Try saying each phoneme separately in the word "length," and then say the word as you normally would by blending the sounds together.

Unlike the /t/p/k/, which intrude in the phonetic context of other consonants, the /j/ and /w/ can intrude between vowels. In the phrase "see it," the /j/ intrudes between the final position vowel of the first word /i/ and the initial vowel /ɪ/ of the word which follows, as in [sijɪt]. The phrase "two apples" provides an example of the intruded /w/, as in [tuwæpəlz]. If the words in the phrases were said separately, the intrusion of /j/ and /w/ would not occur.

Coarticulation

The other type of accommodation is coarticulation. Compared to the major changes in assimilation, coarticulation produces *minor* phonetic changes. Coarticulation occurs as a result of a fast rate of speech. Say the word "moon." Did you notice that your lips were already in position for the /u/ when you were producing the /m/? In Standard American English, vowels are normally produced without nasal resonance except when they appear before or after a nasal consonant, as in [mæ̃n]. This nasality is indicated by the /~/ symbol placed over the sound that has acquired nasal resonance. Symbols that indicate a specific way a phoneme has been produced are termed *diacritics*. This is *narrow transcription,* which uses diacritics to specifically explain how a sound was produced. Contrast this with *broad transcription* which uses only the IPA phoneme symbol to represent a sound.

Frequently used diacritics are listed in Table 15–1. S. Singh and K. Singh (2006) provide an expanded list of diacritics.

Often in conversational speech we extend the duration of a sound, known as *lengthening* or *prolongation.* This occurs frequently when we say two words together, one of which ends in the same sound as the beginning sound of the adjacent word. For example, the phrase "same milk" can be produced as [semːɪlk]. The lengthening diacritic [ː] *follows* the prolonged phoneme.

We can say the phrase "both thumbs" as two separate words, or joined together as in [boθːʌmz]. The diacritic [ː] is used to indicate lengthening. Some examples are provided in Transcription Exercise 15–1.

Table 15–1. Selected Diacritics

Diacritic	Name	Example	Affects	Phoneme(s)
[ʰ]	Aspirated	[pʰost]	Voiceless stops	/p/, /t/, /k/
[˺]	Unreleased	[bæk˺drɔp]	All plosives	/p/, /b/, /t/, /d/, /k/, /g/
[˜]	Nasality	[nõt]	Vowels adjacent to nasals	All vowels & diphthongs
[̥]	Unvoiced	[pr̥ɑɪ]	Follows voiceless consonants	/r/
[̬]	Voiced	[bɛt̬ɚ]	Adjacent to voiced sounds	/t/, /s/
[̩]	Syllabic consonant	[bʌtn̩] [æpl̩]	Lateral and nasals	/l/, /n/, /m/, /ŋ/
[ː]	Prolongation	[dɑːrk]	Emphasized phonemes	Possible with any phonemes

Another change that can occur in speech is *devoicing*. Devoicing occurs when a voiced phoneme becomes unvoiced due to the phonetic environment, but the voiced phoneme does *not* become totally voiceless. The phonetic environment for devoicing is when a voiced phoneme follows an unvoiced phoneme, as in the word "pray" [pr̥e]. The devoicing diacritic is a small circle / ̥ / *under* the devoiced phoneme.

Here is a silly sentence that uses the diacritics discussed in this chapter:

Put these zany dogs in the backdoor of the clean critter kennel.

[pʊtʰ ðizːeñi dɑgz ɪn ði bæk˺ dor ʌv ði kl̥in kr̥ɪt̬ɚ kɛnl̩]

Transcription Exercise 15–1   ◯ **Track: (CD 2, Track 50)**

These words contain examples of: (1) progressive assimilation, (2) regressive assimilation, (3) intrusion, (4) lengthening, and (5) omission.

1. fixed (1)   fɪkst

2. cancel (3)   kæntsəl

3. stop pushing (4)   stɑp ʊʃɪŋ

4. junk (2)   dʒʌŋk

5. pushed (1)   pʊʃt

6. dreamt (3)   drɛmpt

7. go away (5)   ɡo'we

8. wigs (1)   wɪɡz

9. mink (2)   mɪŋk

10. little Lucy (4)   lɪtəl lʊsi

11. fragrance (2)   freɡɹænts

12. stomachs (1)   stʌmɪks

13. kiss her (5)   kɪsɚ

14. comfort (3)   kʌmpfɚt

15. black corn (4)   blæk ɔrn

16. bugs (1)   bʌɡz

17. let me go (5)   lɛmiɡo

18. prince (3)   prɪnts

19. seeds (1)   sidz

20. thin knife (4)   θɪn ɑɪf

STUDY QUESTIONS

1. Define accommodation.

Adjustment or adaptation of speech sounds due to phonetic enviament

2. Define phonetic context.

Phonemes which surrounds a specific speech sound

3. Name two types of accommodation.

Assimilation & Co-articulation

4. What is the difference between progressive and regressive assimilation?

Progressive: occurs left to right. A preceeding phoneme influences the phoneme

5. Why does coarticulation occur?

Occurs as a result of the rapid rate of speech. Produce minor phonetic changes

6. What is a diacritic?

A symbol to indicate a specific way a phoneme was produced

7. What diacritic represents lengthening?

Lengthening diacritic is : or ː

8. What is a phonetic context for devoicing a voiced phoneme?

When voiced phonemes is adjacent to an unvoiced phoneme

9. How do epenthesis and elision differ?

Elision : A phoneme is omitted in a word

Epenthesis : Phoneme can be added.

CHAPTER

16

Dialect Differences

Learning Objectives

After reading this chapter, you will be able to:

1. Define dialect and accent.

2. Name major geographic dialect regions in the United States.

3. List articulation characteristics of African American English, Arabic, Spanish, and Asian speakers.

The focus of this Workbook is phoneme production in Standard American English (SAE). SAE is "accent-free." This is the type of speech you hear when you listen to national broadcasters present the news on television and radio. A *dialect* is a speech or language variation. We refer to an *accent* when we discuss speech that has characteristics of a foreign dialect.

There are several United States dialects representative of various geographic regions including the East, Midwest, and Southern states. Each region has specific variations in pronunciation and language.

Speakers of African American English use specific speech substitutions. These are presented in Table 16–1. Foreign accents in the Arabic, Hispanic, and Asian dialects are included in Tables 16–2, 16–3, and 16–4, respectively.

Dolores Battle (Ed.) offers a detailed discussion of phonological and grammatical differences in numerous languages.

Table 16–1. Characteristics of African American English Articulation and Phonology

Articulation Characteristics	Sample English Utterances
/l/ phoneme lessened or omitted	too'/tool a'ways/always
/r/ phoneme lessened or omitted	doah/door mudah/mother p'otect/protect
f/voiceless "th" substitution at the end or middle of a word	teef/teeth bof/both nufin'/nothing
t/voiceless "th" substitution at the beginning of a word	tink/think tin/thin
d/voiced "th" substitution at the beginning or middle of a word	dis/this broder/brother
v/voiced "th" substitution at the end of a word	breave/breathe smoov/smooth
Consonant cluster reduction	des'/desk res'/rest lef'/left was'/wasp
Differing syllable stress patterns	gui tar/guitar po lice/police Ju ly/July

Source: From *Multicultural Students with Special Language Needs: Practical Strategies for Assessment and Intervention* (Table 4–2, p. 63), by C. Roseberry-McKibbin, 2002, Oceanside, CA: Academic Communication Associates. Copyright 2002 by Academic Communication Associates. Reprinted with permission.

Table 16–2. Articulation and Language Differences Commonly Observed among Arabic Speakers

Articulation Characteristics	Sample English Utterances	
n/ng substitution	son/song	nothin'/nothing
sh/ch substitution	mush/much	shoe/chew
w/v or f/v substitution	west/vest fife/five	Walerie/Valerie abofe/above
t/voiceless "th" or s/voiceless "th" substitution	bat/bath sing/thing	noting/nothing somesing/something
z/voiced "th" substitution	brozer/brother	zese/these
zh/j substitution	zhoke/joke	fuzh/fudge
Retroflex /r/ does not exist	Speakers of Arabic will use a tap or trilled /r/.	
There are no triple consonant clusters in Arabic, so epenthesis may occur	kinduhly/kindly	harduhly/hardly
o/a substitutions	hole/hall	bowl/ball
o/oi substitutions	bowl/boil	foble/foible
uh/ae substitutions	snuck/snack	ruck/rack
i/ɪ substitutions	cheep/chip	sheep/ship
Language Characteristics	**Sample English Utterances**	
Omission of possessives 's and "of"	That Kathy book. The title the story is . . .	
Omission of plurals	She has 5 horse in her stable. He has 3 pen in his pocket.	
Omissions of prepositions	Put your shoes.	
Omission of the form "to be"	She _____ my friend	
Inversion of noun constructs	Let's go to the station gas.	

Source: From *Multicultural Students with Special Language Needs: Practical Strategies for Assessment and Intervention* (Table 9–2, p. 161), by C. Roseberry-McKibbin, 2002, Oceanside, CA: Academic Communication Associates. Copyright 2002 by Academic Communication Associates. Reprinted with permission.

Table 16–3. Articulation Differences Commonly Observed Among Spanish Speakers

Articulation Characteristics	Sample English Utterances
/t, d, n/ may be dentalized (tip of tongue is placed against the back of the upper central incisors)	
Final consonants are often devoiced.	dose/doze
b/v substitution	berry/very
Deaspirated stops (sounds like the speaker is omitting the sound because it is said with little air released).	
ch/sh substitution	chew/shoe
Voiced and voiceless "th" do not exist in Spanish.	dis/this tink/think zat/that
Schwa sound is inserted before word initial consonant clusters.	eskate/skate espend/spend
Words end in vowels only or in just a few consonants (/l, r, n, s, d/).	Speakers may delete many final consonants in English.
When words start with an "h", the "h" is silent.	'old/hold, 'it/hit
/r/ is tapped or trilled (tap /r/ might sound like the tap in the English word "butter")	
"j" (e.g., judge) does not exist in Spanish; speakers may substitute the "y."	Yulie/Julie yoke/joke
The Spanish "s" is produced more frontally than the English "s."	Some speakers may sound like they have frontal lisps.
The ñ is produced as "ny" (e.g., baño is pronounced "bahnyo").	
Spanish has 5 vowels (ɑ,ɛ,i,o,u) and few diphthongs. Thus, Spanish speakers may produce the following vowel substitutions:	
i/ɪ substitution	peeg/pig leetle/little
ɛ/æ, ɑ/æ	pet/pat Stahn, Stan

Source: From *Multicultural Students with Special Language Needs: Practical Strategies for Assessment and Intervention* (Table 5–2, p. 85), by C. Roseberry-McKibbin, 2002, Oceanside, CA: Academic Communication Associates. Copyright 2002 by Academic Communication Associates. Reprinted with permission.

Table 16–4. Articulation Differences Commonly Observed among Asian Speakers

Articulation Characteristics	Sample English Utterances	
In many Asian languages, words end in vowels only or in just a few consonants; speakers may delete many final consonants in English	ste/step ro/robe	li/lid do/dog
Some languages are monosyllabic; speakers may truncate polysyllabic words or emphasize the wrong syllable	efunt/elephant **di**versity/diversity (emphasis on the first syllable)	
Possible devoicing of voiced cognates	beece/bees luff/love	pick/pig crip/crib
r/l confusion	lize/rize	clown/crown
/r/ may be omitted entirely	gull/girl	
Reduction of vowel length in words	Words sound choppy to Americans.	
No voiced or voiceless "th"	dose/those zose/those	tin/thin sin/thin
Epenthesis (addition of "uh" sound in blends or at the end of words)	bulack/black	wooduh/wood
Confusion of "ch" and "sh"	sheep/cheap	beesh/beach
/ae/ does not exist in many Asian languages	block/black	shock/shack
b/v substitutions	base/vase	Beberly/Beverly
v/w substitutions	vork/work	vall/wall

Source: From *Multicultural Students with Special Language Needs: Practical Strategies for Assessment and Intervention* (Table 6–3, p. 109), by C. Roseberry-McKibbin, 2002, Oceanside, CA: Academic Communication Associates. Copyright 2002 by Academic Communication Associates. Reprinted with permission.

STUDY QUESTIONS

1. Standard American English is also identified as:

Accent - free speech

2. Define dialect.

A variation of speech or language

3. Define accent.

Speech characteristic of a foreign dialect

4. Name three dialect regions of the United States.

East, midwest, Southern states

5. According to Roseberry-McKibbin, name three articulation characteristics of African American English.

/t/ substitution for /θ/ in initial position;
Consonant cluster reduction; /r/ phoneme lessened or omitted

6. According to Roseberry-McKibbin, list three articulation characteristics of Spanish speakers.

b/v substitution, schwa inserted before initial consonant cluster, Spanish
"s" produced frontally.

International Phonetic Alphabet

(Revised to 2005)

CONSONANTS (PULMONIC)

	Bilabial	Labiodental	Dental	Alveolar	Postalveolar	Retroflex	Palatal	Velar	Uvular	Pharyngeal	Glottal
Plosive	p b			t d		ʈ ɖ	c ɟ	k g	q ɢ		ʔ
Nasal	m	ɱ		n		ɳ	ɲ	ŋ	ɴ		
Trill	ʙ			r					ʀ		
Tap or Flap				ɾ		ɽ					
Fricative	ɸ β	f v	θ ð	s z	ʃ ʒ	ʂ ʐ	ç ʝ	x ɣ	χ ʁ	ħ ʕ	h ɦ
Lateral fricative				ɬ ɮ							
Approximant		ʋ		ɹ		ɻ	j	ɰ			
Lateral approximant				l		ɭ	ʎ	ʟ			

Where symbols appear in pairs, the one to the right represents a voiced consonant. Shaded areas denote articulations judged impossible.

CONSONANTS (NON-PULMONIC)

Clicks		Voiced implosives		Ejectives	
ʘ	Bilabial	ɓ	Bilabial	ʼ	Examples:
ǀ	Dental	ɗ	Dental/alveolar	pʼ	Bilabial
ǃ	(Post)alveolar	ʄ	Palatal	tʼ	Dental/alveolar
ǂ	Palatoalveolar	ɠ	Velar	kʼ	Velar
ǁ	Alveolar lateral	ʛ	Uvular	sʼ	Alveolar fricative

VOWELS

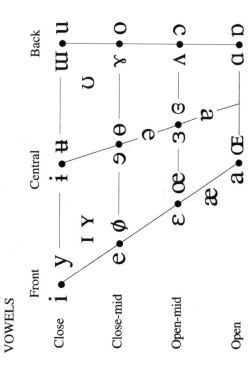

Where symbols appear in pairs, the one to the right represents a rounded vowel.

OTHER SYMBOLS

ʍ Voiceless labial-velar fricative	ɕ ʑ Alveolo-palatal fricatives
w Voiced labial-velar approximant	ɺ Alveolar lateral flap
ɥ Voiced labial-palatal approximant	ɧ Simultaneous ʃ and x
ʜ Voiceless epiglottal fricative	
ʢ Voiced epiglottal fricative	Affricates and double articulations can be represented by two symbols joined by a tie bar if necessary.
ʡ Epiglottal plosive	k͡p t͡s

SUPRASEGMENTALS

ˈ	Primary stress	ˌfoʊnəˈtɪʃən
ˌ	Secondary stress	
ː	Long	eː
ˑ	Half-long	eˑ
˘	Extra-short	ĕ
ǀ	Minor (foot) group	
‖	Major (intonation) group	
.	Syllable break	ɹi.ækt
‿	Linking (absence of a break)	

TONES AND WORD ACCENTS

LEVEL			CONTOUR		
e̋ or ꜛ	Extra high		ě or ꜛ	Rising	
é ꜛ	High		ê ꜜ	Falling	
ē ꜛ	Mid		e᷄ ꜛ	High rising	
è ꜛ	Low		e᷅ ꜛ	Low rising	
ȅ ꜛ	Extra low		e᷈ ꜛ	Rising-falling	
ꜜ	Downstep		↗	Global rise	
ꜛ	Upstep		↘	Global fall	

DIACRITICS Diacritics may be placed above a symbol with a descender, e.g. ŋ̊

̥	Voiceless	n̥ d̥	̤	Breathy voiced	b̤ a̤	̪	Dental	t̪ d̪
̬	Voiced	s̬ t̬	̰	Creaky voiced	b̰ a̰	̺	Apical	t̺ d̺
ʰ	Aspirated	tʰ dʰ	̼	Linguolabial	t̼ d̼	̻	Laminal	t̻ d̻
̹	More rounded	ɔ̹	ʷ	Labialized	tʷ dʷ	̃	Nasalized	ẽ
̜	Less rounded	ɔ̜	ʲ	Palatalized	tʲ dʲ	ⁿ	Nasal release	dⁿ
̟	Advanced	u̟	ˠ	Velarized	tˠ dˠ	ˡ	Lateral release	dˡ
̠	Retracted	e̠	ˤ	Pharyngealized	tˤ dˤ	̚	No audible release	d̚
̈	Centralized	ë	̴	Velarized or pharyngealized	ɫ			
̽	Mid-centralized	e̽	̝	Raised	e̝ (ɹ̝ = voiced alveolar fricative)			
̩	Syllabic	n̩	̞	Lowered	e̞ (β̞ = voiced bilabial approximant)			
̯	Non-syllabic	e̯	̘	Advanced Tongue Root	e̘			
˞	Rhoticity	ɚ a˞	̙	Retracted Tongue Root	e̙			

Answers to Exercises

Chapter 2

Transcription Exercise 2–1
Track: (CD 1, Track 2)

Number of Sounds		Transcription
2	1. gnaw	[nɔ]
3	2. shape	[ʃep]
5	3. cousin	[kʌzɪn]
4	4. leisure	[liʒɚ]
3	5. tongue	[tʌŋ]
2	6. who	[hu]
4	7. rather	[ræðɚ]
3	8. tough	[tʌf]
3	9. kneel	[nil]
3	10. ax	[æks]
7	11. cinnamon	[sɪnʌmɪn]
3	12. wrap	[ræp]
4	13. raked	[rekt]
3	14. sight	[saɪt]
5	15. phoneme	[fonim]

Transcription Exercise 2–2
Track: (CD 1, Track 3)

[præktɪs ɛvɝi de]

Transcription Exercise 2–3
Track: (CD 1, Track 4)

Consonants	Vowels
1. /k/	7. /u/
2. /ŋ/	8. /i/
3. /dʒ/	9. /o/
4. /f/	10. /ɝ/
5. /j/	11. /e/
6. /z/	12. /a/

Exercise 2–A

Syllable Division	# Syllables
1. co-da	2
2. nu-cle-us	3
3. vow-el	2
4. syl-la-ble	3
5. rhyme	1
6. i-ni-tial	3
7. me-di-al	3
8. fi-nal	2
9. blend	1
10. clus-ter	2
11. ar-rest-ing	3
12. re-leas-ing	3
13. con-so-nant	3
14. or-thog-ra-phy	4

15. pound	1
16. wig-gle	2
17. in-tel-li-gence	4
18. math-e-mat-i-cal	5
19. cen-ti-me-ter	4
20. choc-o-late	3

Exercise 2–B
Syllable Shapes

1. V C   ash
   æ ʃ

2. C C V C   crash
   k r æ ʃ

3. C C C V C   splash
   s p l æ ʃ

4. V C C V C   eastern
   i s t ɚ n

5. C C V C   green
   g r i n

6. C C V   three
   θ r i

7. C C V C   preach
   p r i tʃ

8. C C C V C   scream
   s k r i m

9. C C V C   frame
   f r e m

10. C V C C V C V C   phosphorus
    f a s f o r ə s

Exercise 2–C

1. Brachyceratops
   C C V C V C V C V C V C C
   b r a k i s ɛ r a t a p s

2. Corythosaurus
   C V C V C V C V C V C
   k o r i θ o s a r ə s

3. Dilophosaurus
   C V C V C V C V C V C
   d ɪ l o f o s a r ə s

4. Microceratops
   C V C C V C V C V C V C C
   m aɪ k r o s ɛ r a t a p s

5. Pachyrhinosaurus
C V C V C V C V C V C V
p æ k i r aɪ n o s a r ə s

6. Pentaceratops
C V C C V C V C V C V C C
p ɛ n t ə s ɛ r a t a p s

7. Triceratops
C C V C V C V C V C C
t r aɪ s ɛ r a t a p s

8. Brachiosaurus
C C V C V V C V C V C
b r a k i o s a r ə s

9. Epachthosaurus
V C V C C V C V C V C
ɛ p æ k θ o s a r ə s

10. Heterodontosaurus
C V C V V C V C C V C V C V C
h ɛ t ɚ o d a n t o s a r ə s

Chapter 3

Exercises 3–A through 3–E.

Answers are in **bold** print

Exercise 3–A Manner of articulation: Stop-Consonants

1. **B**lack**b**ir**d**
2. **D**ay **T**ri**pp**er
3. **G**e**t** Bac**k**
4. **P**a**p**er**b**ack Wri**t**er
5. **T**icke**t** to Ri**d**e
6. A Har**d** **D**ay's Nigh**t**
7. I **G**o**t** to Fin**d** My **B**a**b**y
8. I'll **B**e **B**ac**k**
9. Come an**d** **G**e**t** I**t**
10. Le**t** I**t** **B**e

Exercise 3–B Manner of articulation: Nasals

1. If I **N**eeded So**m**eo**n**e
2. Lady **M**ado**nn**a
3. Le**n**d **M**e Your Co**m**b
4. **M**a**gg**ie **M**ae
5. Pe**nn**y La**n**e
6. Su**n** Ki**ng**
7. Tax**m**a**n**
8. I'**m** O**n**ly Sleepi**ng**
9. Tip of **M**y To**ng**ue
10. **M**ail**m**a**n**, Bri**ng** **M**e **N**o **M**ore Blues

Exercise 3–C Manner of articulation: Fricatives

1. Another Girl
2. Strawberry Fields Forever
3. Dizzy Miss Lizzy
4. Good Day Sunshine
5. Here Comes the Sun
6. I Saw Her Standing There
7. If I Fell
8. I've Just Seen a Face
9. Lucy in the Sky with Diamonds
10. She Came in Through the Bathroom Window

Exercise 3–D Manner of articulation: Liquids and Glides

1. Eleanor Rigby
2. Lovely Rita
3. Yellow Submarine
4. Words of Love
5. Young Blood
6. Ballad of John and Yoko
7. Watching Rainbows
8. Winston's Walk
9. Yesterday
10. Run for your Life

Exercise 3–E Manner of articulation: Affricates

1. Act Naturally
2. Julia
3. Magical Mystery Tour
4. Mother Nature's Son
5. Norwegian Wood
6. Blue Jay Way
7. Baby You're a Rich Man
8. Chains
9. Her Majesty
10. Hey Jude

Chapter 4

Transcription Exercise 4–1

1. [fon]
2. [splɪt]   M
3. [hɪkəp]   F
4. [gofɚ]
5. [ʃapɪŋ]   M
6. [prɛsɪdɛnt]   I
7. [pɛpɚmɪnt]   I & M
8. [numætɪk]

9. [əpɛnd]   M
10. [pæmflɪt]   I

/p/ Transcription Exercise 4–2
Track: (CD 1, Track 6)

1. [paɪn]
2. [dip]
3. [əˈpoz]
4. [kep]
5. [ˈpepɚ]
6. [sɪp]
7. [ples]
8. [hɛlp]
9. [pæk]

/b/ Transcription Exercise 4–3
Track: (CD 1, Track 7)

1. [hʌmbəl]   M
2. [rɪbɪn]   M
3. [bilebɚ]   I & M
4. [pʌblɪk]   M
5. [bɚbæŋk]   I & M
6. [θʌm]
7. [prob]   F
8. [hælɪbʌt]   M
9. [brok]   I
10. [tumston]

/b/ Transcription Exercise 4–4
Track: (CD 1, Track 8)

1. [bæd]
2. [tʌb]
3. [ˈbebi]
4. [braɪt]
5. [ˈræbɪt]
6. [ˈnobədi]
7. [bɑm]
8. [kɔb]
9. [kɝb]

/p/ and /b/ Crossword

Across   Down
1. [pɑliwɑg]   1. [pɛbəl]
3. [kʌb]   2. [lipɪŋ]
4. [pʌmps]
5. [brɪŋ]

/t/ Transcription Exercise 4–5
Track: (CD 1, Track 9)

1. [kɔt]   F
2. [wɪsəl]

3. [tuwɪʃɪn]   I
4. [taɪm]   I
5. [tɛntətɪv]   I & M
6. [tortijə]   I & M
7. [wɑtʃt]   F
8. [ʃæle]
9. [tɛrɪtori]   I & M
10. [moʃən]

t/ Transcription Exercise 4–6
Track: (CD 1, Track 10)

1. [tʌb]
2. [kʌt]
3. [ˈɪntu]
4. [ˈʌntɪl]
5. [twɪn]
6. [kot]
7. [ˈrotet]
8. [taɪm]
9. [nɛst]

Glottal Stop Transcription Exercise 4–7
Track: (CD 1, Track 11)

1. [ˈdulɪtəl]   [dulɪʔl̩]
2. [ˈmɪtən]   [mɪʔn̩]
3. [ˈfaʊntən]   [faʊnʔn̩]
4. [ˈpætənt]   [pæʔn̩t]
5. [ˈhɪltən]   [hɪlʔn̩]
6. [ˈbʌtən]   [bʌʔn̩]
7. [ˈlætən]   [læʔn̩]
8. [ˈkɔtən]   [kɔʔn̩]
9. [ˈbɪtən]   [bɪʔn̩]
10. [ˈmoltən]   [molʔn̩]

Voiced /t/ Transcription Exercise 4–8
Track: (CD 1, Track 12)

1. [bɛˈtɚ]   [ˈbɛt̬ɚ]
2. [hɔˈtɚ]   [ˈhɔt̬ɚ]
3. [bæˈtəl]   [ˈbæt̬əl]
4. [mæˈtɚ]   [ˈmæt̬ɚ]
5. [æˈtəm]   [ˈæt̬əm]
6. [bʌˈtɚ]   [ˈbʌt̬ɚ]
7. [keˈtɚ]   [ˈket̬ɚ]
8. [kwoˈtə]   [ˈkwot̬ə]
9. [tʃiˈtɪd]   [ˈtʃit̬ɪd]
10. [duˈti]   [ˈdut̬i]

/d/ Transcription Exercise 4–9
Track: (CD 1, Track 13)

1. [hɛdʒ]
2. [hæŋkɚtʃɪf]

3. [mæpt]
4. [dɛdɪnd]   I & M & F
5. [dɛked]   I & F
6. [pɔɪntɛd] F
7. [ædɪŋ]   M
8. [mɪdɪjəl] M
9. [drɛd]   I & F
10. [dɪmænd] I & F

/d/ Transcription Exercise 4–10
Track: (CD 1, Track 14)

1. [do]
2. [ˈkʌndɪʃən]
3. [ju̯zd]
4. [dɪʃ]
5. [ˈmɛdo]
6. [sænd]
7. [dwɛl]
8. [ˈwʌndɚ]
9. [ˈtʃendʒd]

/t/ and /d/ Crossword Puzzle

Across	Down
1. [dɛf]	1. [daɪmz]
2. [dɪziz]	2. [dituɚ]
3. [detə]	3. [dat]

/k/ Transcription Exercise 4–11
Track: (CD 1, Track 15)

1. [sɛntɪmitɚ]
2. [pike]   M
3. [kwortɛt]   I
4. [tɛkst]   M
5. [braŋkaɪtɪs] M
6. [ɪmpɛkəbəl] M
7. [krɪtɪk]   I & F
8. [bækek]   M & F
9. [naɪt]
10. [tokvɪl]   M

/k/ Transcription Exercise 4–12
Track: (CD 1, Track 16)

1. [bæk]
2. [kaʊnt]
3. [tɪk]
4. [ˈbæskɪt]
5. [kek]
6. [krim]
7. [ˈstakɪŋ]
8. [əˈkras]
9. [marˈki]

/g/ Transcription Exercise 4–13
Track: (CD 1, Track 17)

1. [dʒɛntəl]
2. [garbɪdʒ] I
3. [næt]
4. [ɛgnag]   M & F
5. [ɛgzɪst]   M
6. [gaʊdʒ]   I
7. [læf]
8. [gɚtrud]   I
9. [lɪŋgɚ]   M
10. [dɪdʒɪt]

/g/ Transcription Exercise 4–14
Track: (CD 1, Track 18)

1. [gan]
2. [ˈwɪgəl]
3. [ˈhʌŋgri]
4. [bɛg]
5. [dɔg]
6. [grin]
7. [veg]
8. [glʌv]
9. [ˈgrɪdəl]

/k/ and /g/ Crossword Puzzle

Across	Down
2. [ʃʊgɚ]	1. [jogɚt]
3. [brɛkfɛst]	3. [bekən]
5. [kɔfi]	4. [ɛgz]
6. [næpkɪn]	

Stop-Consonant Transcription Exercise 4–15
Track: (CD 1, Track 19)

1. [ˈpɚpɪtret]
2. [ˈbʌkɪt]
3. [ˈklepat]
4. [drapt]
5. [pop]
6. [datudat]
7. [ˈkʌpkek]
8. [ˈbebid]
9. [ˈdɛdbolt]
10. [kot]
11. [ˈpʌgodə]
12. [ˈbɚdbik]
13. [fɪkst]
14. [ˈlæptap]
15. [ˈgæbi]
16. [ˈdagtæg]
17. [ˈbækʌp]
18. [ˈtogə]
19. [pɔkɪtbʊk]
20. [kɛpt]

Chapter 5

/m/ Transcription Exercise 5–1
Track: (CD 1, Track 20)

1. [mɚmed]   I & M
2. [daɪm]   F

3. [pɑm] F
4. [mʌm] I & F
5. [kæzəm] F
6. [mɪnɪmʌm] I & M & F
7. [mɛmbrən] I & M
8. [hæmɚ] M
9. [skwɝm] F
10. [ɛmpɑɪjɚ] M

/m/ Transcription Exercise 5–2
Track: (CD 1, Track 21)

1. [mɑɪt]
2. [læmp]
3. [mit]
4. [tim]
5. ['kæmɚə]
6. [mɑlt]
7. ['rændəm]
8. [hɑrm]
9. [smɛl]

/n/ Transcription Exercise 5–3
Track: (CD 1, Track 22)

1. [næpsæk] I
2. [kɛnəl] M
3. [nɑnsɛnᵗs] I & M
4. [zon] F
5. [næʃ] I
6. [numætɪk] I
7. [nun] I & F
8. [nom] I
9. [bɪgɪnɚ] M
10. [sɛvɪntin] F

/n/ Transcription Exercise 5–4
Track: (CD 1, Track 23)

1. ['tɛnɪs]
2. ['kæbɪn]
3. ['nɔɪzi]
4. ['kʌnɛri]
5. ['nɑtɪkəl]
6. ['vɑɪolɪn]
7. ['hændi]
8. ['pænəl]
9. ['nɑɪlɑn]

/ŋ/ Transcription Exercise 5–5
Track: (CD 1, Track 24)

1. [mʌŋki] M
2. [sɪŋɪŋ] M & F
3. [kɪŋdʌm] M
4. [ʌrendʒ]

5. [ilɑŋgɛt] M
6. [rɔŋ] F
7. [dʒɪŋgəl] M
8. [lɛŋkθ] M
9. [fɛŋz] M
10. [spʌndʒ]

/ŋ/ Transcription Exercise 5–6
Track: (CD 1, Track 25)

1. ['bɔŋgo]
2. ['strɑŋgli]
3. ['hɑŋkɑŋ]
4. [wɪŋ]
5. [tʌŋ]
6. ['ʃɪŋgəl]
7. ['dɑɪnɪŋ]
8. [fɛŋ]
9. ['sevɪŋz]

/m/ /n/ and /ŋ/ Crossword Puzzle

Across
1. [nɑɪn]
3. [kɪŋdəm]
4. [numonjə]

Down
1. [næpkɪn]
2. [stim]

Nasal Consonant Transcription Exercise 5–7
Track: (CD 1, Track 26)

1. ['nezəl]
2. ['mɑnjumɛntəl]
3. [ə'mʌŋ]
4. ['rɛmnɪnt]
5. [nɑmɪnet]
6. ['fɛmɪnɪn]
7. ['lɛmoned]
8. ['mornɪŋ]
9. ['tʃɪmni]
10. [mi'tɪŋ]
11. ['kʌntenɪŋ]
12. ['mɪŋglɪŋ]
13. ['mɛmbrɛn]
14. ['mʌni]
15. ['næni]
16. ['mɝeŋ]
17. ['mɑʊntɪn]
18. ['numɛrɪkəl]
19. [sɪnə'mʌn]
20. ['munbɪm]

Transcription Exercise 5–8
Track: (CD 1, Track 27)

		Formal Speech	Casual Speech
1.	cabin	[kæbɪn]	[kæbm̩]
2.	medal	[mɛdəl]	[mɛdl̩]
3.	redden	[rɛdɪn]	[rɛdn̩]
4.	ribbon	[rɪbɪn]	[rɪbm̩]
5.	blacken	[blækɪn]	[blækŋ̩]
6.	panel	[pænəl]	[pænl̩]
7.	milking	[mɪlkɪŋ]	[mɪlkŋ̩]
8.	garden	[gɑrdɪn]	[gɑrdn̩]
9.	broken	[brokɪn]	[brokŋ̩]
10.	open	[opɪn]	[opm̩]

Chapter 6

/f/ Transcription Exercise 6–1
Track: (CD 1, Track 28)

1. [fɑsforəs]   I & M
2. [pæmflɪt]   M
3. [dʒɝæf]   F
4. [foto]   I
5. [fɪftin]   I & M
6. [dʒosɪf]   F
7. [sfɪrɪkəl]   M
8. [manogræf]   F
9. [flʌfi]   I & M
10. [fonəgræf]   I & F

/f/ Transcription Exercise 6–2
Track: (CD 1, Track 29)

1. [fʌn]
2. [biˈfor]
3. [ˈfɪftin]
4. [frɑst]
5. [ˈkɔfi]
6. [lif]
7. [læf]
8. [flot]
9. [ɪf]

/v/ Transcription Exercise 6–3
Track: (CD 1, Track 30)

1. [vɪndɪktɪv]   I & F
2. [waɪf]
3. [ʃɛvran]   M
4. [wivɚ]   F
5. [ʌv]   F
6. [laɪfsevɪŋ]   M
7. [nɛvɚ]   M
8. [waɪvz]   M
9. [vɛrɪfaɪ]   I
10. [stov]   F

/v/ Transcription Exercise 6–4
Track: (CD 1, Track 31)

1. [vaɪn]
2. [ˈvɛlvɪt]
3. [ˈovɚ]
4. [ˈvɛri]
5. [ˈɪnvaɪt]
6. [lɪv]
7. [ˈvælju]
8. [wivɚ]
9. [muv]

/f/ and /v/ Crossword Puzzle

Across   Down
1. [kæfin]   1. [kævɪti]
4. [ves]   2. [fɛstɪvəl]
5. [flɪp]   3. [notɪfaɪ]

/s/ Transcription Exercise 6–5
Track: (CD 1, Track 32)

1. [sɪti]   I
2. [ʃevz]
3. [disɛptɪv]   M
4. [blɪnts]   F
5. [juʒjul]
6. [æksɪz]   M
7. [breslɪt]   M
8. [aɪlɪnd]
9. [sudo]   I
10. [braŋks]   F

/s/ Transcription Exercise 6–6
Track: (CD 1, Track 33)

1. [ɛls]
2. [əˈslip]
3. [suˈpirijɚ]
4. [ˈbesɪn]
5. [ˈɪstɚ]
6. [ˈsidɚ]
7. [æsks]
8. [ˈsændəl]
9. [blæst]

/z/ Transcription Exercise 6–7
Track: (CD 1, Track 34)

1. [kɪdz]   F
2. [zɑr]   I
3. [tʃiz]   F
4. [abzɝv]   M
5. [bɪznɪs]   M
6. [nɑzəl]   M
7. [prɛzɪnt]   M
8. [ɪz]   F
9. [siʒɚ]
10. [babslɛdz]   F

/z/ Transcription Exercise 6–8
Track: (CD 1, Track 35)

1. [ˈbɪzi]
2. [ˈvɪzɪt]
3. [ˈzɝkan]
4. [ˈwizəl]

5. [siz]
6. ['zɪnijə]
7. [ðoz]
8. ['zukini]
9. [gɪvz]

/s/ and /z/ Crossword Puzzle

Across
3. [zɪp]
4. [sɪzəl]
5. [soldʒɚ]

Down
1. [sups]
2. [zil]
3. [zoro]
5. [sizənz]

Fricative Consonant Transcription Exercise 6–9
Track: (CD 1, Track 37)

1. ['fɛstɪv]
2. [swɪs]
3. ['vɛsəl]
4. ['fænsɪfʊl]
5. ['mizəlz]
6. [zɛst]
7. ['vɪvɪd]
8. ['ɛkspɛnsɪv]
9. ['bɪznɪsɪz]
10. [for'gɪv]
11. ['sopsʌdz]
12. ['fæsɪn]
13. [skwiz]
14. ['sɪzɚz]
15. ['farməsi]
16. ['stivɪn]
17. [vaɪs]
18. ['swɪtzɚlænd]
19. [sef'tɪ]
20. [sɪ'vɪljən]

/θ/ I-M-F Table Transcription Exercise 6–10
Track: (CD 1, Track 38)

1. [ɛnθuzijæst]   M
2. [θɚzde]   I
3. [θɪðɚ]   I
4. [ilɪzʌbɛθ]   F
5. [θɚti θɚd]   I & M
6. [gaθɪk]   M
7. [kʌθidrəl]   M
8. [θru]   I
9. [ænɪsθiʒʌ]   M
10. [zinɪθ]   F

/θ/ Transcription Exercise 6–11
Track: (CD 1, Track 39)

1. [θɪn]
2. ['bɚθde]
3. [wɪdθ]
4. [tiθ]
5. [θro]
6. ['ɪniθɪŋ]
7. [norθ]
8. ['nʌθɪŋ]
9. [θɔ]

/ð/ I-M-F Table Transcription Exercise 6–12
Track: (CD 1, Track 40)

1. [ðɛm]   I
2. [kloð]   F
3. [hɛðɚ]   M
4. [rɪðəm]   M
5. [tiθ]
6. [norθ]
7. [wɛðɚ]   M
8. [θaɪ]
9. [norðɚn]   M
10. [wɛðɚ]   M

/ð/ Transcription Exercise 6–13
Track: (CD 1, Track 41)

1. [ðɪs]
2. ['iðɚ]
3. [ðɛr]
4. ['faðɚ]
5. [sɪð]
6. [ðo]
7. ['mʌðɚ]
8. [tɪð]
9. [smuð]

"th" Transcription Exercise 6–14
Track: (CD 1, Track 42)

1. ð	11. ð	21. θ
2. ð	12. θ	22. θ
3. θ	13. θ	23. θ
4. θ	14. ð	24. ð
5. ð	15. ð	25. θ
6. ð	16. θ	26. ð
7. θ	17. ð	27. ð
8. ð	18. ð	28. ð
9. θ	19. ð	29. ð
10. ð	20. θ	30. θ

/θ/ and /ð/ Crossword Puzzle

Across
1. [faðɚ]
2. [ðoz]
3. [mʌðɚz]
4. [θɪn]
6. [rɪðəm]

Down
1. [fɛðɚz]
3. [mɛθadɪk]
5. [norθ]

Interdental Consonant Transcription Exercise 6–15
Track: (CD 1, Track 43)

1. [baɪk'ʌθɔn]
2. [wadz'wɚθ]
3. [saʊθistɚn]
4. ['ʌrɪθmətɪk]

5. [sɛvəntinθ]
6. [ˈθrɛtɪn]
7. [ˌʌndɚgroθ]
8. [sʌðɚnmost]
9. [θʌndɚˈbɚd]
10. [ˈplɪməθ]
11. [ruθlesli]
12. [wɪðɚspun]
13. [ˈhartθrab]
14. [ˈwɚði]
15. [ˈθraɪvɪŋ]
16. [ənˈʌðɚ]
17. [mɛθadɪk]
18. [ˈθaʔlɛs]
19. [ˈhʌndrɛθ]
20. [ˈlɛðɚ]

/h/ Transcription Exercise 6–16
Track: (CD 1, Track 44)

1. [hum]   I
2. [rihɚs]   M
3. [hɪtʃhaɪk]   I & M
4. [ʌnholsəm]   M
5. [hoze]   I
6. [ɪnhel]   M
7. [hɪləmanstɚ]   I
8. [hæbɪtæt]   I
9. [mʌhagəni]   M
10. [ɛkshələʃən] M

/h/ Transcription Exercise 6–17
Track: (CD 1, Track 45)

1. [hɛft]
2. [ˈharbɚ]
3. [moˈhɛr]
4. [ˈʌphɪl]
5. [hʌm]
6. [ˈɪnhɛrɪt]
7. [ˈrihɚs]
8. [ˈhɚmɪt]
9. [ˈʌnhʊk]

/ʍ/ I-M-F Table Transcription Exercise 6–18
Track: (CD 1, Track 46)

1. [ʍil]   I
2. [kʍin]   M
3. [sʍɛr]   M
4. [ʍaɪ]   I
5. [sʍed]   M
6. [ʍɛr]   I
7. [holʍit]   M
8. [wɛr]
9. [wægɪn]
10. [skʍɛr]   M

/ʍ/ Transcription Exercise 6–19
Track: (CD 1, Track 47)

1. [ʍɪm]
2. [ˈovɚʍɛlm]

3. [ʍɪp]
4. [ˈtʍɛntɪ]
5. [ʃʍa]
6. [ʍaɪt]
7. [ˈsʌmʍɛr]
8. [ˈʍɛðɚ]
9. [ʍorf]

/h/ and /hw/ Transcription Exercise 6–20
Track: (CD 1, Track 48)

1. [ˈhɛdʒhag]
2. [sʍed]
3. [ʍɚl]
4. [hum]
5. [sʍe]
6. [ˈwahu]
7. [ʍaɪn]
8. [hændˈʃek]
9. [her]
10. [ʍɪf]
11. [hu]
12. [ˈʍæmɪ]
13. [holharˈtɪd]
14. [ʍɛr]
15. [ˈpɪnʍil]
16. [hɪm]
17. [ˈpɚsʍed]
18. [ʍɪsəl]
19. [ohaɪo]
20. [huz]

/ʃ/ Transcription Exercise 6–21
Track: (CD 1, Track 49)

1. [kʌndɪʃən]   M
2. [ʌʃɚ]   M
3. [tɪʃju]   M
4. [broʃɚ]   M
5. [ʃɪfan]   I
6. [ɪnɪʃəl]   M
7. [trɛʒɚ]
8. [lɪkorɪʃ]   F
9. [krieʃən]   M
10. [ʃubrʌʃ]   I & F

/ʃ/ Transcription Exercise 6–22
Track: (CD 1, Track 50)

1. [ʃu]
2. [ˈmʌstæʃ]
3. [ˈoʃən]
4. [ˈɪnʃɚ]
5. [wɪʃ]
6. [ʃɪp]
7. [ˈrɛlɪʃ]
8. [ʃek]
9. [ˈfæʃən]

/ʒ/ Transcription Exercise 6–23
Track: (CD 1, Track 51)

1. [vɪʒɪn]   M
2. [ʌfeʒə]   M
3. [gʌraʒ]   F

4. [steʃən]
5. [trɛʒɚ]   M
6. [pɝʒə]   M
7. [kloʒɚ]   M
8. [ruʒ]   F
9. [kʌmpoʒɚ]   M
10. [tɛləvɪʒən] M

/ʒ/ Transcription Exercise 6–24
Track: (CD 1, Track 52)

1. ['rɛʒim]
2. [loʒ]
3. ['plɛʒɚ]
4. ['dɪvɪʒɪn]
5. ['juʒuəl]
6. ['kʌlɪʒɪn]
7. [beʒ]
8. ['kolɑʒ]
9. [kæʒul]

/ʃ/ and /ʒ/ Crossword Puzzle

Across
1. [vekeʃən]
3. [liʒɚ]
4. [ʌfeʒə]
6. [ʃʌn]

Down
2. [kʌlɪʒən]
5. [fɪʃ]

Chapter 7

/tʃ/ Transcription Exercise 7–1
Track: (CD 1, Track 53)

1. [ʃɛf]
2. [hætʃɪt]   M
3. [pɪtʃ]   F
4. [broʃɚ]
5. [kord]
6. [kʌltʃɚ]   M
7. [ek]
8. [mʌʃin]
9. [tʃɝtʃ]   I & F
10. [fjutʃɚ]   M

/tʃ/ Transcription Exercise 7–2
Track: (CD 1, Track 54)

1. [tʃɪn]
2. ['pitʃɪz]
3. [wɪtʃ]
4. [tʃiz]
5. [lʌntʃ]
6. ['titʃɚ]

7. ['tʃɪldrɛn]
8. [skatʃ]
9. ['fɝnətʃɚ]

/dʒ/ Transcription Exercise 7–3
Track: (CD 1, Track 55)

1. [gʌrɑdʒ]   F
2. [bʌdʒɪt]   M
3. [dʒɪndʒɚ]   I & M
4. [dʌndʒən]   M
5. [dʒʌmp]   I
6. [ɛdʒjukeʃən] M
7. [dʒɛstʃɚ]   I
8. [vɔɪjɪdʒ]   F
9. ['ɪndʒɪn]   M
10. [splɝdʒ]   F

/dʒ/ Transcription Exercise 7–4
Track: (CD 1, Track 56)

1. [dʒʌŋk]
2. [ɛn'dʒɔɪ]
3. [ɝdʒd]
4. ['vɪdʒəl]
5. [wedʒ]
6. [dʒɛm]
7. ['dʒʌmbo]
8. ['kɑlədʒɪn]
9. [fʌdʒ]

/tʃ/ and /dʒ/ Crossword Puzzle

Across
2. [endʒəlz]
3. [ridʒɔɪs]
5. [pritʃɚz]

Down
1. [klɝdʒi]
4. [samz]

Fricative and Affricate Consonant Transcription Exercise 7–5
Track: (CD 1, Track 57)

1. ['ʃuʃaɪn]
2. ['daɪdʒɛstʃən]
3. ['kʌnfjuʒɪn]
4. ['antɝɑʒ]
5. [ægrɪ'kʌltʃɚ]
6. [vaɪ'veʃəs]
7. ['sæbətɑʒ]
8. [ɛn'tʃæntɪd]
9. [dʒek]
10. [ʃɪptuʃor]
11. ['stedʒkotʃ]
12. ['tʃaɪldɪʃ]
13. ['hadʒpadʒ]
14. [pɛriʒən]
15. ['sʌgdʒɛstʃən]
16. ['tʃɪntʃɪlə]
17. [kolɛkʃən]
18. [fortʃənɪt]
19. [bjutɪʃən]
20. [vɪʒjulaɪz]

Chapter 8

/w/ Transcription Exercise 8–1
Track: (CD 1, Track 58)

1. [wʌnts]   I
2. [wɪdo]   I
3. [gwɑm]   M
4. [twaɪs]   M
5. [ɪgwɑnə]   M
6. [ʌɛr]
7. [kiwi]   M
8. [kʌɛstʃɪn]
9. [wɪlo]   I
10. [ɛŋgwɪʃ]   M

/w/ Transcription Exercise 8–2
Track: (CD 1, Track 59)

1. [wæks]
2. ['dʒægwɑr]
3. [bi'wɛr]
4. [swɛl]
5. ['wʌndɚ]
6. [kwin]
7. ['forwɚd]
8. [twɪn]
9. [wɛt]

/j/ Transcription Exercise 8–3
Track: (CD 1, Track 60)

1. [ɪndʒɛkt]
2. [rɔɪjəl]   M
3. [jɛt]   I
4. [zɪljən]   M
5. [bʌnjən]   M
6. [spænjəl]   M
7. [jojo]   I & M
8. [lejɛt]   M
9. [fɪgjɚ]   M
10. [kaɪjoti]   M

/j/ Transcription Exercise 8–4
Track: (CD 1, Track 61)

1. [jor]
2. [bi'jɑnd]
3. [jild]
4. [pʌ'paɪjə]
5. ['jɑndɚ]
6. [fʌmɪljɚ]
7. [jɑrn]
8. ['bɪljʌn]
9. [jɛs]

/l/ Transcription Exercise 8–5
Track: (CD 1, Track 62)

1. [mɔl]   F
2. [lɪnolijəm]   I & M
3. [wel]   F
4. [æpəl]   F
5. [fɛlo]   M
6. [kævz]
7. [lʌləbaɪ]   I & M
8. [flotɪlə]   M
9. [hɛlm]   M
10. [soʃəbəl]   F

/l/ Transcription Exercise 8–6
Track: (CD 1, Track 63)

1. ['lʌki]
2. ['lɛmən]
3. [klaʊn]
4. ['sændəl]
5. ['goldən]
6. [ɛls]
7. ['braɪdəl]
8. [fli]
9. ['liɑn]

/r/ Transcription Exercise 8–7
Track: (CD 1, Track 64)

1. [ræp]   I
2. [raɪ]   I
3. [skɑr]   F
4. [riport]   I & M
5. [rʌbɚ]   M
6. [wordrob]   M
7. [raɪ]   I
8. [gɑrdɪn]   M
9. [bifor]   F
10. [dir]   F

/r/ Transcription Exercise 8–8
Track: (CD 1, Track 65)

1. [raɪt]
2. [ɪm'prɛs]
3. [ri'dus]
4. ['sɑri]
5. [raɪm]
6. ['ɔlrɛdi]
7. [tʃɛr]
8. [rʌb]
9. [bɑr]

/ir/ Transcription Exercise 8–9
Track: (CD 1, Track 66)

1. [spir]   F
2. [wird]   M
3. [siriz]   M
4. [stir]   F
5. [pɛr]   F
6. [firs]   M
7. [irʌ]   I
8. [kʌrir]   F
9. [mɝθ]
10. [waɪjɚ]

/ɛr/ Transcription Exercise 8–10
Track: (CD 1, Track 67)

1. [stɛr]   F
2. [skwɛr]   F
3. [bɛrəl]   M
4. [wɛr]   F
5. [trelɚ]
6. [stɛr]   F
7. [pɝl]
8. [tʃɛr]   F
9. [bɛr]   F
10. [kɛrəmɛl]   M

/ɑr/ Transcription Exercise 8–11
Track: (CD 1, Track 68)

1. [hɑrt]   M
2. [stɑr]   F
3. [sɑrdʒɪnt]   M
4. [fɑrs]   M
5. [kɛrɪdʒ]
6. [stɛr]
7. [mɛri]
8. [mʌrin]
9. [pɑrti]   M
10. [kɑrbʌn]   M

/or/ Transcription Exercise 8–12
Track: (CD 1, Track 69)

1. [forθ]   M
2. [kʍort]   M
3. [pɑrlɚ]
4. [worʃ]   M
5. [sor]   F
6. [wort]   M
7. [rumɚ]
8. [kort]   M
9. [por]   F
10. [wɝld]

/j/, /l/, and /r/ Crossword Puzzle

Across	Down
2. [jɛlo]	1. [til]
4. [roz]	3. [orɪndʒ]
5. [dʒʌŋgəlgrin]	6. [lævɪndɚ]
7. [vaɪolɛt]	
8. [mərun]	

Vowel plus r Transcription Exercise 8–13
Track: (CD 1, Track 70)

1. ['irmɑrk]   11. [spɑrs]
2. ['kɛrworn]   12. ['ɑrdvɑrk]
3. [or]   13. [dʒir]
4. [spirz]   14. [bor]
5. ['kɑrport]   15. ['forskʍɛr]
6. [ʃir]   16. [fɑrs]
7. ['hɑrdwɛr]   17. [kors]
8. [dɑrt]   18. [smirz]
9. [for'lorn]   19. [stɑrtʃ]
10. [rɛr]   20. [bɛr]

Oral Resonant Consonant Transcription Exercise 8–14
Track: (CD 1, Track 71)

1. [jok]   11. ['redijetɚ]
2. [dworf]   12. ['kʍaɪjɪtli]
3. ['liwe]   13. ['væljɛnt]
4. ['domɪnjʌn]   14. ['frikʍɛntsi]
5. ['kʍɪbəl]   15. ['lɔɪjɚ]
6. ['lɑrsɪni]   16. ['wewɚd]
7. ['jɝenijəm]   17. ['jolandʌ]
8. [ɪləstret]   18. ['stæljʌnz]
9. ['ræli]   19. ['rɛsəl]
10. ['sɔɪjɚ]   20. [jɔn]

Chapter 10

/i/ Transcription Exercise 10–1
Track: (CD 2, Track 1)

1. [jɛs]
2. [livɪŋ]   M
3. [il]   I
4. [θivz]   M
5. [pipəl]   M
6. [tʃipɪn]   M
7. [kiʃ]   M
8. [strit]   M
9. [hilɪks]   M
10. [haɪjɚ]

/i/ Transcription Exercise 10–2
Track: (CD 2, Track 2)

1. [it]
2. [kip]
3. [did]
4. [ki]
5. [bik]
6. [pik]
7. [bit]
8. [ti]
9. [dip]

/ɪ/ Transcription Exercise 10–3
Track: (CD 2, Track 3)

1. [maɪld]
2. [ɪt]   I
3. [pɪksi]   M
4. [bɪljən]   M
5. [faɪn]
6. [gɪlt]   M
7. [vɪlɪn]   M
8. [sɪnsiɚ]   M
9. [lɪmpf]   M
10. [fɪn]   M

/ɪ/ Transcription Exercise 10–4
Track: (CD 2, Track 4)

1. [kɪk]
2. [gɪg]
3. [bɪld]
4. [tɪk]
5. [ɪt]
6. [bɪt]
7. [pɪk]
8. [kɪd]
9. [bɪg]

/ɛ/ Transcription Exercise 10–5
Track: (CD 2, Track 5)

1. [ɛntel]   I
2. [pɛŋgwɪn] M
3. [bɛl]   M
4. [maɪld]
5. [jɛs]   M
6. [ɛlf]   I
7. [gæŋ]
8. [ɛθɪk]   I
9. [gɛs]   M
10. [dʒɛləs] M

/ɛ/ Transcription Exercise 10–6
Track: (CD 2, Track 6)

1. [mɛld]
2. [ɛnd]
3. [dɛl]
4. [dɛn]
5. [lɛd]
6. [nɛl]
7. [dɛnts]
8. [slɛd]
9. [ɛtʃ]

/e/ Transcription Exercise 10–7
Track: (CD 2, Track 7)

1. [ekorn]   I
2. [sle]   F
3. [ven]   M
4. [daɪl]
5. [liʒɚ]
6. [gen]   M
7. [bæg]
8. [le]   F
9. [əten]   M
10. [rendir] M

/e/ Transcription Exercise 10–8
Track: (CD 2, Track 8)

1. [ves]
2. [stez]
3. [zen]
4. [et]
5. [fez]
6. [test]
7. [fes]
8. [ʃev]
9. [fet]

/æ/ Transcription Exercise 10–9
Track: (CD 2, Track 9)

1. [ædvænts] I & M
2. [pæn]   M
3. [ænt]   I
4. [mɑl]
5. [pen]
6. [dæmpnɪs] M
7. [kwæk]   M
8. [kæsked]   M
9. [mæθ]   M
10. [wɛnt]

/æ/ Transcription Exercise 10–10
Track: (CD 2, Track 10)

1. [sæʃ]
2. [fæst]
3. [æʃ]
4. [stæf]
5. [væt]
6. [ʃæft]
7. [tæt]
8. [æz]
9. [sæv]

/i/, /ɪ/, /ɛ/, /e/, /æ/, and /w/ Crossword Puzzle

Across
1. [wɛbstɚ]
2. [wɪnstʌn]
4. [len]
5. [mɛri]

Down
1. [wɪn]
2. [wɪljʌm]
3. [tɪm]
6. [ʃilʌ]

Front Vowel Transcription Exercise 10–11
Track: (CD 2, Track 11)

1. [flem]
2. ['æli]
3. [bi'liv]
4. [re'zɪn]
5. [wik'de]
6. ['rilæks]
7. [æsk]
8. ['pipəl]
9. [rɛmnɪnt]
10. [ren]
11. ['dʒɪmnɪst]
12. ['eprɪn]
13. ['nemsek]
14. ['bɪzi]
15. ['kæfin]
16. ['wɪmɪn]
17. ['hɛdek]
18. [pliz]
19. ['bɪskɪt]
20. ['ɛldɪst]

Chapter 11

/ə/ Transcription Exercise 11–1
Track: (CD 2, Track 12)

1. [əhɛd]   I
2. [rətæn]   M
3. [məʃin]   M
4. [bətan]   M
5. [kʌbanə]   F
6. [tubə]   F
7. [vænɪlə]   F
8. [əgri]   I
9. [bəfe]   M
10. [kəkun]   M

/ə/ Transcription Exercise 11–2
Track: (CD 2, Track 13)

1. [gə'lor]
2. [sə'port]
3. [ə'lon]
4. [kəm'poz]
5. [kən'don]
6. [pə'trol]
7. [rə'por]
8. [ə'ʃor]
9. [lə'gun]

/ə/ Crossword Puzzle

Across
4. [səpoz]
5. [kəkun]
6. [ləgun]

Down
1. [pəpus]
2. [gəzəl]
3. [əpan]

/ʌ/ Transcription Exercise 11–3
Track: (CD 2, Track 14)

1. [ʌv]   I
2. [tʃʌg]   M
3. [wʌn]   M
4. [ʌnkʌt]   I & M
5. [wʌz]   M
6. [jʌŋ]   M
7. [rʌst]   M
8. [ʌp]   I
9. [wʌn]   M
10. [rust]

/ʌ/ Transcription Exercise 11–4
Track: (CD 2, Track 15)

1. [ʌvɪn]
2. [tʌtʃ]
3. [θʌm]
4. [bʌm]
5. [tʌn]
6. [pʌn]
7. [mʌt]
8. [kʌd]
9. [nʌt]

/ʌ/ Crossword Puzzle

Across
3. [ʌnglud]
6. [ʃʌt]

Down
1. [dʌst]
2. [hʌʃ]
4. [gʌmbo]
5. [dʌk]

/ɚ/ Transcription Exercise 11–5
Track: (CD 2, Track 16)

1. [æktɚ]   M
2. [ɝnɚ]   F
3. [nɝd]

4. [ʃʊgɚ]   F
5. [eŋgɚ]   F
6. [nebɚ]   F
7. [kritʃɚ]   F
8. [kɝtɪn]
9. [glæmɚ]   F
10. [pepɚ]   F

/ɚ/ Transcription Exercises 11–6
Track: (CD 2, Track 17)

1. [ˈnetʃɚ]
2. [ˈmedʒɚ]
3. [ˈbekɚ]
4. [ˈrezɚ]
5. [ˈletɚ]
6. [ˈpesɚ]
7. [ˈfeljɚ]
8. [ˈnebɚ]
9. [ˈsefɚ]

/ɚ/ Crossword Puzzle

Across
3. [flaʊwɚ]
4. [læntɚn]

Down
1. [ɛvɚ]
2. [ɛfɚt]
4. [lidɚ]
5. [nɛvɚ]

/ɝ/ Transcription Exercise 11–7
Track: (CD 2, Track 18)

1. [ɝb]   M
2. [wɝst]   M
3. [slɝ]   F
4. [tʃɝp]   M
5. [sɝdʒɪn]   M
6. [ɝn]   I
7. [pɝtʃəs]   M
8. [ɝn]   I
9. [tɝtəl]   M
10. [mɝtəl]   M

/ɝ/ Transcription Exercise 11–8
Track: (CD 2, Track 19)

1. [ɝdʒ]
2. [vɝb]
3. [bɝθ]
4. [θɝd]
5. [dɝdʒ]
6. [bɝ]
7. [gɝθ]
8. [dʒɝm]
9. [ɝθ]

/ɝ/ Crossword Puzzle

Across
2. [ɝbəl]
4. [θɝsti]
6. [nɝsmed]

Down
1. [bɝst]
3. [zɝkan]
5. [θɝd]

Central Vowels Transcription Exercise 11–9
Track: (CD 2, Track 20)

1. [hæmbɚgɚ]
2. [sʌdz]
3. [kɝn]
4. [ˈkʌvɚ]
5. [ʌˈkɚ]
6. [ˈfɝvɚ]
7. [ˈʌndʌn]
8. [ˈirdrʌm]
9. [ˈmɝmɚ]
10. [əˈwaɪl]
11. [ˈtɝnɚ]
12. [kʌnˈfɝm]
13. [ˈbʌzɚ]
14. [ˈmʌtʃɚ]
15. [ˈbʌfɚ]
16. [tʃɝp]
17. [sɝdʒ]
18. [vɝs]
19. [sʌbˈmɝdʒ]
20. [ˈmɝdʒɚ]

/ə/ Transcription Exercise 11–11
Track: (CD 2, Track 22)

1. cousin   cousin   [ˈkʌzən]
2. illness   illness   [ˈɪlnəs]
3. distant   distant   [ˈdɪstənt]
4. promise   promise   [ˈpraməs]
5. palace   palace   [ˈpæləs]
6. socket   socket   [ˈsakət]
7. disease   disease   [ˈdəziz]
8. escape   escape   [ˈəskep]
9. contain   contain   [kənˈten]
10. divide   divide   [dəˈvaɪd]

/ʌ/ Transcription Exercise 11–12
Track: (CD 2, Track 23)

1. gulf   [gʌlf]
2. dust   [dʌst]
3. dumb   [dʌm]
4. fuzz   [fʌz]
5. putt   [pʌt]
6. plus   [plʌs]
7. lug   [lʌg]
8. stuck   [stʌk]
9. crumb   [krʌm]
10. plum   [plʌm]

/ɝ/ Transcription Exercise 11–13
Track: (CD 2, Track 24)

1. clerk   [klɝk]
2. first   [fɝst]
3. heard   [hɝd]
4. fur   [fɝ]

5. cursed   [kɝst]
6. shirk   [ʃɝk]
7. were   [wɝ]
8. whirl   [wɝl]
9. per   [pɝ]
10. curl   [kɝl]

/ʌ/ɝ/ Transcription Exercise 11–14
Track: (CD 2, Track 25)

1. bun	[bʌn]	burn	[bɝn]
2. shuck	[ʃʌk]	shirk	[ʃɝk]
3. buzz	[bʌz]	burns	[bɝnz]
4. hut	[hʌt]	hurt	[hɝt]
5. shut	[ʃʌt]	shirt	[ʃɝt]
6. cut	[kʌt]	curt	[kɝt]
7. luck	[lʌk]	lurk	[lɝk]
8. putt	[pʌt]	pert	[pɝt]
9. bust	[bʌst]	burst	[bɝst]
10. hub	[hʌb]	Herb	[hɝb]

/ɚ/ Transcription Exercise 11–15
Track: (CD 2, Track 26)

1. plumber   ['plʌmɚ]
2. other   ['ʌðɚ]
3. cluster   ['klʌstɚ]
4. ulcer   ['ʌlsɚ]
5. buffer   ['bʌfɚ]
6. butler   ['bʌtlɚ]
7. plunger   ['plʌndʒɚ]
8. rubber   ['rʌbɚ]
9. southern   ['sʌðɚn]
10. sculpture ['skʌlptʃɚ]

Chapter 12

/u/ Transcription Exercise 12–1
Track: (CD 2, Track 27)

1. [nudəl]   M
2. [du]   F
3. [du]   F
4. [ʃʊd]
5. [uz]   I
6. [sut]   M
7. [butik]   M
8. [ful]   M
9. [duk]   M
10. [tu]   F

/u/ Transcription Exercise 12–2
Track: (CD 2, Track 28)

1. [rul]
2. [su]

3. [lus]
4. [ru]
5. [lup]
6. [flu]
7. [slup]
8. [pul]
9. [ful]

/ʊ/ Transcription Exercise 12–3
Track: (CD 2, Track 29)

1. [fʊl]   M
2. [ʊps]   I
3. [wʊlf]   M
4. [mʌt]
5. [sʊt]   M
6. [guf]
7. [wʊps]   M
8. [ʃʊgɚ]   M
9. [fʊtstul]   M
10. [hʊd]   M

/ʊ/ Transcription Exercise 12–4
Track: (CD 2, Track 30)

1. [kʊk]
2. [wʊl]
3. [fʊt]
4. [wʊd]
5. [lʊk]
6. [wʊlf]
7. [fʊl]
8. [kʊd]
9. [nʊk]

/o/ Transcription Exercise 12–5
Track: (CD 2, Track 31)

1. [old]   I
2. [mut]
3. [so]   F
4. [loʃən]   M
5. [mo]   F
6. [hu]
7. [kolə]   M
8. [tost]   M
9. [bol]   M
10. [matʃo]   F

/o/ Transcription Exercise 12–6
Track: (CD 2, Track 32)

1. [not]
2. [ton]
3. [on]
4. [tot]

5. [no]
6. [ot]
7. [hon]
8. [no]
9. [o]

/ɔ/ Transcription Exercise 12–7
Track: (CD 2, Track 33)

1. [ɔl]	I
2. [θɔŋ]	M
3. [sɔs]	M
4. [ɔ]	I
5. [ʃwɔ]	F
6. [mɔθ]	M
7. [pɔ]	F
8. [skwɔ]	F
9. [pɔ]	F
10. [θɔt]	M

/ɔ/ Transcription Exercise 12–8
Track: (CD 2, Track 34)

1. [sɔt]
2. ['bɔdi]
3. [rɔt]
4. [prɔn]
5. [kɔl]
6. [tɔt]
7. [θɔt]
8. [vɔlt]
9. [lɔfʊl]

/a/ Transcription Exercise 12–9
Track: (CD 2, Track 35)

1. [pasʈə]	M
2. [amənd]	I
3. [spa]	F
4. [lantʃ]	M
5. [ʒanrə]	M
6. [jat]	M
7. [akwə]	I
8. [lʌntʃ]	
9. [ʃwa]	F
10. [antre]	I

/a/ Transcription Exercise 12–10
Track: (CD 2, Track 36)

1. [a]
2. [nat]
3. [ha]
4. [jat]
5. [tat]

6. [jan]
7. [hant]
8. [tat]
9. [ant]

/u/, /ʊ/, /o/, /ɔ/, and /a/ Crossword Puzzle

Across	Down
3. [ɔfʊl]	1. [θɔŋ]
5. [laŋ]	2. [fʊt]
6. [to]	4. [lo]
7. [sok]	5. [lus]

Back Vowel Transcription Exercise 12–11
Track: (CD 2, Track 37)

1. ['kupan]	11. ['kʊkbʊk]
2. [hʊk]	12. ['bostfʊl]
3. ['ankor]	13. ['fʊtstul]
4. [ha'θorn]	14. ['horsʃu]
5. ['nuzrum]	15. [fɔt]
6. ['tako]	16. ['dormrum]
7. ['jojo]	17. [frut]
8. ['ɔfʊl]	18. ['maθbɔl]
9. [jat]	19. [sok]
10. [lalipap]	20. ['θɔtfʊl]

Chapter 13

/aɪ/ Transcription Exercise 13–1
Track: (CD 2, Track 38)

1. [aɪlɪnd]	I
2. [aɪ]	I
3. [gaɪ]	F
4. [maɪnəs]	M
5. [daɪl]	M
6. [raɪm]	M
7. [swit]	
8. [haɪ]	F
9. [nis]	
10. [braɪd]	M

/aɪ/ Transcription Exercise 13–2
Track: (CD 2, Track 39)

1. [baɪ]
2. ['saɪdɚ]
3. [haɪt]
4. ['faɪsti]
5. [slaɪs]
6. [taɪm]
7. [raɪt]
8. [saɪ]
9. [raɪm]

/aʊ/ Transcription Exercise 13–3
Track: (CD 2, Track 40)

1. [aʊtʃ]   I
2. [lɑn]
3. [kaʊwɚd]   M
4. [vaʊwəl]   M
5. [haʊ]   F
6. [tɑfi]
7. [ʃaʊt]   M
8. [no]
9. [laʊndʒ]   M
10. [haʊs]   M

/aʊ/ Transcription Exercise 13–4
Track: (CD 2, Track 41)

1. [aʊst]
2. [traʊt]
3. ['gaʊdʒɪŋ]
4. [praʊwəl]
5. ['tʃaʊdɚ]
6. ['haʊshold]
7. [baʊnd]
8. [laʊs]
9. [baʊ]

/ɔɪ/ Transcription Exercise 13–5
Track: (CD 2, Track 42)

1. [kɔɪ]   F
2. [tʃɔɪs]   M
3. [taʊn]
4. [dʒɔɪn]   M
5. [saɪfɚ]
6. [mɔɪst]   M
7. [mɪst]
8. [bɔɪjɛnt]   M
9. [dʒʒus]
10. [spɔɪl]   M

/ɔɪ/ Transcription Exercise 13–6
Track: (CD 2, Track 43)

1. ['hɔɪstɪŋ]
2. ['kɔɪld]
3. ['dɛstrɔɪ]
4. [fɔɪlz]
5. ['lɔɪtɚ]
6. ['vɔɪsɪŋ]
7. [tɔɪ]
8. [ɛks'plɔɪt]
9. [ə'vɔɪd]

/ju/ Transcription Exercise 13–7
Track: (CD 2, Track 44)

1. [fju]   F
2. [junjən]   I
3. [bjuti]   M
4. [kjut]   M
5. [pju]   F
6. [juz]   I
7. [hjudʒ]   M
8. [ful]
9. [hjumɚ]   M
10. [hulə]

/ju/ Transcription Exercise 13–8
Track: (CD 2, Track 45)

1. [juk]
2. ['fjuʃə]
3. ['mjuzɪk]
4. [hjudʒ]
5. ['mjutɪnt]
6. ['pjupəl]
7. [spjud]
8. [bjut]
9. [fjum]

Diphthong Crossword Puzzle

Across
1. [mɔɪst]
3. [kju]
4. [daʊn]
6. [naɪn]

Down
1. [mju]
2. [spɔɪld]
5. [naʊn]
7. [aɪsaɪt]

Diphthong Transcription Exercise 13–9
Track: (CD 2, Track 46)

1. ['faʊndri]
2. [dʒɔɪn]
3. ['jukɑn]
4. [braɪn]
5. [tɔɪl]
6. [dʒænjuwɛri]
7. [aʊst]
8. ['jukəleli]
9. [mɔɪst]
10. ['æmjulɛt]
11. [paʊt]
12. [baɪt]
13. [naʊn]
14. [nɔɪz]
15. ['fraʊnɪŋ]
16. [aɪ]
17. [kʌntrɪbjutɚ]
18. [ɔɪŋk]
19. [maɪm]
20. ['braʊniz]

Chapter 14

Transcription Exercise 14–2 (#6–10)
Track: (CD 2, Track 48)

Stressed syllable is in **bold** print.

Noun	Verb
6. 'record	6. re'**cord**
7. 'invalid	7. in'**valid**
8. 'desert	8. de'**sert**
9. 'refuse	9. re'**fuse**
10. '**present**	10. pre'**sent**

Transcription Exercise 14–3
Track: (CD 2, Track 49)

	Syllable Division	Number of Syllables
1. 'licorice	lic-or-ice	(3)
2. in'gredient	in-gre-di-ent	(4)
3. 'crying	cry-ing	(2)
4. a'nother	a-noth-er	(3)
5. 'audible	au-di-ble	(3)
6. hi'larious	hi-lar-i-ous	(4)
7. se'curity	se-cu-ri-ty	(4)
8. com'puter	com-put-er	(3)
9. 'saxophone	sax-o-phone	(3)
10. 'bigger	big-ger	(2)
11. 'pleasure	plea-sure	(2)
12. aggra'vation	ag-gra-va-tion	(4)
13. 'aftermath	af-ter-math	(3)
14. 'resource	re-source	(2)
15. pre'pare	pre-pare	(2)
16. 'liberal	lib-er-al	(3)
17. water'melon	wa-ter-mel-on	(4)
18. gener'ation	gen-er-a-tion	(4)
19. e'vaporate	e-vap-o-rate	(4)
20. 'public	pub-lic	(2)

Chapter 15

Transcription Exercise 15–1
Track: (CD 2, Track 50)

1. [fɪkst]	11. ['fregrænts]
2. ['kæntsəl]	12. ['stʌmɪks]
3. [stapːʊʃɪŋ]	13. [kɪsˈɝ]
4. [dʒʌŋk]	14. ['kʌmpfɚt]
5. [pʊʃt]	15. [blækːorn]
6. [drɛmpt]	16. [bʌgz]
7. [goˈwe]	17. [lɛmigo]
8. [wɪgz]	18. [prɪnts]
9. [mɪŋk]	19. [sidz]
10. [lɪtəlːusi]	20. [θɪnːaɪf]

Chapter 4 Word Search #1: /p/ and /b/

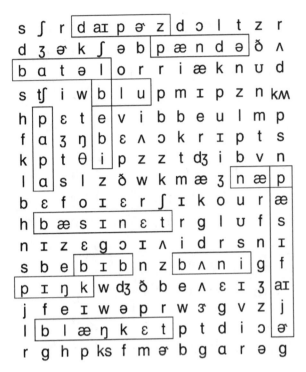

Chapter 4 Word Search #2:
/t/, /d/, /k/, and /g/

Chapter 5 Word Search #3: /m/ and /n/

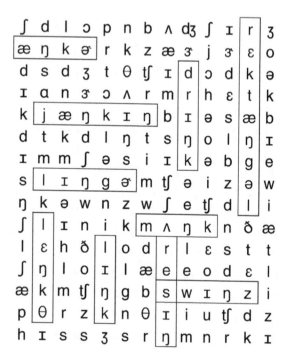

Chapter 5 Word Search #4: /ŋ/

Chapter 6 Word Search #5: /f/ and /v/

Chapter 6 Word Search #6: /s/ and /z/

Chapter 6 Word Search #7: /θ/ and /ð/

```
g  t  k  ɛ  l  v  b  ʌ  k  b  m  s
ɝ  ʒ  p  æ  θ  h  e  b  m  ɛ  θ  aʊ
k  p  o  r  ɛ  e  ð  ɛ  ɪ  d  ð  d
l  p  θ  t  m  v  m  ɛ  o  e  æ  m
o  o  r  æ  ð  b  a  ð  ɚ  l  n  a
ð  k  ɛ  n  p  f  θ  l  d  t  t  m
e  θ  d  d  e  n  e  ð  ɚ  p  æ  æ
v  n  k  m  g  tʃ æ  t  e  k  n  θ
æ  ɚ  ð  g  r  θ  ɪ  ŋ  l  l  r  ɪ
θ  n  t  æ  ɝ  ʒ  θ  ɚ  z  a  t  ɛ
r  g  n  ð  v  d  r  w  ɪ  θ  aʊ t
j  b  o  ɚ  k  h  ɪ  b  s  e  t  i
ə  æ  g  m  s  aʊ θ  a  l  m  ɛ  g
t  θ  t  θ  p  z  n  r  i  æ  n  k
```

Chapter 6 Word Search #8: /ʃ/ and /ʒ/

```
ʃ  æ  l  o  k  ʃ  s  z  n  æ  aɪ p
d  d  d  p  r  r  ɪ  ɪ  k  n  g  ɔ
ɪ  l  ʌ  æ  o  ɪ  t  k  θ  o  l  ɪ
k  n  k  n  j  m  i  l  ɪ  ʃ  k  ə
d  r  m  ʃ  ɪ  p  s  s  ŋ  ə  r  n
ɪ  a  ə  d  u  r  m  l  s  n  a  i
s  d  ɪ  s  n  o  ə  z  z  d  f  ʒ
n  s  n  d  t  f  ɪ  ʃ  k  r  ɚ  ə
ʃ  o  l  e  θ  e  ð  ɔ  o  u  j  k
i  m  m  l  w  z  ʃ  ə  l  ʃ  æ  d
ʃ  a  r  k  d  i  l  ə  h  w  b  o
l  i  s  p  r  o  n  ð  n  ɛ  r  l
æ  t  r  ɛ  ʒ  ɚ  tʃ ɛ  s  t  t  æ
p  m  k  l  æ  m  ʃ  ɛ  l  b  m  b
h  ɪ  tʃ u  o  d  ɔ  e  s  ɚ  ɪ  ʒ
d  k  ɪ  z  b  ʌ  r  l  ɛ  m  n  r
```

Chapter 7 Word Search #9: /tʃ/ and /dʒ/

```
k  p  a  s  s  a  g  e  z  e  dʒ i  p  b  r  j  m  ɛ
n  k  w  tʃ k  v  u  i  tʃ kʍ o  f  z  g  j  r  s  n
d  b  t  s  i  ə  b  ɛ  ks tʃ e  n  dʒ n  u  tʃ v  d
j  s  p  k  æ  z  h  v  s  t  o  h  i  g  m  v  ɪ  z
m  j  æ  h  u  h  a  h  w  n  ɛ  w  f  dʒ p  r  l  t
p  æ  d  v  ɛ  n  tʃ ɚ  k  θ  u  p  ʌ  z  s  p  ɪ  m
m  e  c  z  v  l  ʒ  p  æ  s  ɪ  dʒ ɛ  p  o  k  dʒ n
m  m  s  h  p  b  f  o  g  s  t  ʃ  dʒ h  w  g  g  ŋ
g  a  dʒ ɪ  ŋ  k  s  s  t  z  æ  l  ɪ  o  e  æ  ʌ  a
t  v  ɪ  f  k  g  θ  c  d  ʃ  l  k  u  j  h  s  u  ʍ
v  d  l  i  æ  o  n  d  dʒ h  l  m  f  v  ʌ  s  ə  j
t  f  ɛ  r  ʌ  i  ʒ  r  n  ʒ  f  æ  æ  z  f  n  s  r
r  b  r  ɪ  dʒ ɛ  z  l  ɪ  m  z  d  dʒ p  ɛ  ɪ  b  z
j  b  w  e  ɪ  f  ŋ  ɪ  l  n  m  ɪ  v  ks h  i  ʃ  ʌ
i  w  o  o  k  v  ɛ  u  æ  ŋ  d  k  m  u  w  tʃ h  ɛ
l  n  h  r  ʃ  ð  n  ɚ  tʃ c  o  v  h  n  j  p  ʒ  p
ʊ  z  s  ɪ  n  tʃ ə  p  f  o  s  p  ɛ  h  t  i  tʃ t
z  h  t  u  t  h  ʍ  b  v  u  n  ʒ  l  m  r  w  dʒ d
```

Chapter 8 Word Search #10: /w/

```
g  w  a  n  t  a  n  a  m  o  b  e
ʃ  ɛ  w  e  r  s  ð  r  d  b  ʃ  s
s  a  b  s  ð  ŋ  l  r  j  o  m  h
æ  p  v  ɪ  v  o  ʃ  tʃ b  m  n  aʊ
n  a  k  v  f  w  a  t  ɚ  l  u  w
w  p  r  ɪ  i  ʌ  ə  j  v  w  θ  ɪ
a  w  ɝ  l  d  w  o  c  r  w  ʌ  t
n  tʃ ɪ  w  p  b  t  d  k  g  s  z
h  a  b  ɔ  r  æ  p  e  p  k  w  ɚ
ɪ  ʒ  n  r  e  dʒ ɚ  u  o  θ  o  ð
l  ʃ  æ  u  t  b  n  z  b  l  a  j
r  w  ɛ  p  ə  n  e  w  l  d  j  ɝ
d  p  ɛ  t  e  v  i  h  b  w  e  m
p  æ  n  d  p  aʊ w  ɚ  ʊ  c  l  u
ɚ  z  d  ɔ  l  t  r  d  ʒ  r  v  i
```

Chapter 8 Word Search #11: Vowel + r

Chapter 10 Word Search #13: Front Vowels

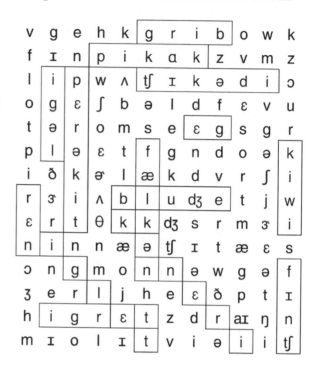

Chapter 8 Word Search #12: /j/, /l/, and /r/

Chapter 11 Word Search #14: /ɚ/ and /ɝ/

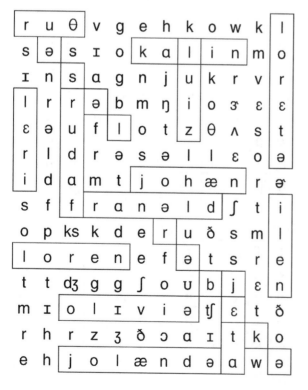

Chapter 12 Word Search #15: Back Vowels   **Chapter 13 Word Search #16: Diphthongs**

Chapter 12 grid:

```
s  ʃ  r  a  dʒ ɚ  d  ɔ  l  t  r  i  z  v  m  f  ʍ
dʒ ʒ  ɚ  k  j  u  ə  b  a  a  z  ð  ʌ  ɝ  a  n  ɪ
b  ʌ  dʒ ɔ  z  j  o  r  a  r  i  r  ɛ  v  æ  ʌ  k
ʊ  k  p  s  θ  i  s  a  ɛ  t  æ  ɪ  w  m  n  u  d
l  r  ɛ  k  h  n  dʒ b  u  g  s  z  ð  e  d  o  r
w  ʌ  p  z  s  u  z  ɪ  n  l  u  tʃ i  w  p  m  ɔ
ɪ  p  v  t  ð  i  z  n  z  ɪ  l  o  p  h  a  d  m
ŋ  æ  k  s  ʃ  u  k  ʍ  h  f  n  v  ɛ  o  b  k  f  a
k  s  g  t  o  θ  p  u  m  p  ʒ  o  p  s  ɝ  ɪ  g
l  ɪ  u  æ  l  j  h  d  u  g  ŋ  m  n  p  t  l  r
b  w  f  e  w  o  k  ʍ  tʃ ɪ  o  u  e  i  l  z  ɔ
h  a  i  ə  ʌ  g  a  r  θ  b  r  u  k  s  o  g  s
n  k  w  tʃ æ  z  ʌ  z  h  t  w  b  v  u  n  ʒ  d
s  ʍ  ɪ  k  d  r  ɔ  ə  g  r  ɔ  j  h  i  g  t
j  r  u  p  ɔ  l  ɚ  f  ɛ  ɝ  b  f  dʒ u  w  e  l
l  ks ɪ  dʒ o  r  dʒ b  u  ʃ  t  s  f  z  r  s  n
```

Chapter 13 grid:

```
s  ʃ  r  d  o  n  p  ɚ  r  ɔ  t  t  v
h  aɪ æ  k  s  v  ju z  p  n  ə  v  ʌ
d  s  t  ə  ɛ  ɛ  c  b  ɔ  ɔɪ n  r  d
b  h  i  n  b  w  w  r  b  s  z  f  k
s  aʊ ɛ  t  k  z  ʌ  u  ʊ  t  i  h  p
h  s  aʊ θ  b  aʊ n  d  m  ɚ  b  ju s
f  p  ʒ  m  ɪ  g  z  i  m  ʒ  u  m  n
k  æ  w  aɪ l  d  f  aʊ l  æ  ʊ  ɚ  p
l  ɛ  t  n  æ  k  h  ʌ  ɪ  k  s  n  æ
b  b  s  θ  p  ə  r  z  d  p  i  g  s
h  ɪ  f  ŋ  s  ɔɪ l  v  z  ɔɪ v  ʒ  z
n  ju æ  l  ks dʒ t  ʃ  e  z  i  z  f
s  b  z  f  ju ʃ  ə  t  r  w  g  ɔ  aɪ
o  ɪ  k  aʊ tʃ g  j  r  æ  m  ɑ  ɚ  j
```

Answers to Study Questions

Chapter 1

1. To accurately transcribe the speech of a client and so that another professional can identify how speech sounds were produced.

2. Greek.

3. A sound/symbol system used to represent the sounds of all languages.

4. Must learn a new sound/symbol system for the majority of the IPA vowels.

5. Study of speech sounds.

6. a. Organs that produce speech and their function (physiological phonetics).
   b. Physical properties of speech sounds (acoustic phonetics).
   c. Process of speech sound perception (perceptual phonetics).

7. a. /ʃ/ b. /θ/ /ð/ c. /ŋ/ d. /i/ e. /ə/ f. /æ/

8. Phonemic (broad transcription) does not use diacritic marks to specify how a speech sound was produced (narrow transcription).

Chapter 2

1. "C"—Consonant "V"—Vowel

2. Initial: First sound heard.
   Medial: Sound in middle of a word.
   Final: Last sound heard at end of the word.

3. Prevocalic: Consonant preceding a vowel.
   Intervocalic: Consonant occurring between two vowels.
   Postvocalic: Consonant after a vowel.

4. Nucleus: Vowel of a syllable.
   Onset: Consonant that releases the nucleus of a syllable.
   Coda: Consonant after a vowel.

5. A vowel, diphthong or syllabic consonant.

6. Open syllable: "bee"
   Closed syllable: "beet"

7. "scrape"   C C C V C
                 s k r e p

8. How a word is spelled.

Chapter 3

1. Survival function.

2. Phonation Articulation Respiration Resonation

3. Place: *Where* the speech sound is produced.
   Manner: *How* the speech sound is produced.

4. In the nasal cavity.

5. Adducted: Vocal folds *close* and vibrate.
   Abducted: Vocal folds *open* and do not vibrate.

6. a. lips
   b. glottis
   c. tongue and upper and lower teeth
   d. alveolar ridge
   e. hard palate
   f. velum or soft palate

7. Two or three consonants in the same syllable.

8. Obstruent: Obstruction of vocal tract.
   Sonorant: Open channel not blocked.

Chapter 4

1. Air is stopped in oral cavity; air is released.

2. Vocal folds adduct to hold air in glottis; vocal folds abduct to open and release air.

3. Only voicing differs.

4. Tongue tip and blade briefly contact, or flaps, against upper Alveolar ridge.

5. Glottal stop/voiced /t/ and alveolar flap.

6. a. /g/ b. /d/ c. /b/

7. a. Allophonic variation of /t/ and /k/
   b. NOT written as a question mark
   c. When glottal stop is followed by /n/, a syllabic /n/ is used.

Chapter 5

1. /m/n/ŋ/

2. /m/ is a bilabial (produced with both lips), /n/ is a lingua-alveolar, /ŋ/ is a lingua-velar.

3. Made in the same *place* as another phoneme.

4. A consonant that acts like a vowel.

5. Formal: Used in a formal setting such as giving a speech.
Casual: Speaking with friends or family.

6. Homorganic relationships: /n/t,d,s,z
/m/b,p   /ŋ/k,g

7. A (ˌ) is placed below the syllabic consonant. Example: /m̩/

Chapter 6

1. Both phonemes are unvoiced when produced in isolation.

2. Glottis.

3. Tongue position not relevant.

4. Tongue tip up: At upper alveolar ridge behind central incisors.
Tongue tip down: Contacts lower incisors behind lower alveolar ridge.

5. Interdental: Breath stream emitted between central incisors.
Lateral: Breath stream emitted around the sides of the tongue.

6. Theta.

7. Sides contact upper molars; tip at lower central incisors; front of tongue elevates toward hard palate.

Chapter 7

1. /t/ and /ʃ/ for /tʃ/ /d/ and /ʒ/ for /dʒ/.

2. Stop-fricatives.

3. Produced with an obstructed breath stream.

4. /t/d/ or omitted.

5. /tʃ/   a. children   b. ketchup
/dʒ/   a. region   b. joke

6. To eliminate confusing the symbols as two separate phonemes.

Chapter 8

1. Approximation of the articulators.

2. Can occur between a word ending in /i/ adjacent to a word beginning with /ɪ/ when the words are spoken as one utterance. Example: "she is" [ʃijɪz]

3. /kw/ or /kʍ/.

4. Lateral airflow around the sides of the tongue.

5. a. Robert
   b. carrot
   c. fairy
   d. sparkle
   e. portrait

6. Position of closeness of articulators which causes some constriction.

Chapter 9

1. A syllable must contain a vowel or diphthong.

2. Tongue does not make contact with a specific articulator for closure.

3. The vocal tract is mostly unobstructed.

4. Monophthong: Single sound (one vowel).
Diphthong: Two sounds (two vowels).

5. Provides reference for tongue position.

6. Vertical: Height of tongue.
Horizontal: Tongue advancement.

7. A tense tongue requires muscular tension at root of tongue; a lax tongue requires less muscular tension at root of tongue.

Chapter 10

1. Unrounded, slightly retracted.

2. Short "i."

3. /æ/ also called "ash."

4. squid myth built

5. /æ/

6. /ɛ/

7. /eɪ/

Chapter 11

1. /ɚ/ /ɝ/

2. Middle of the oral cavity.

3. a. /ɝ/ produced with greater duration
   b. /ɝ/ can form a syllable
   c. tongue moves toward the /r/ consonant
   d. /r/ is voiceless following a voiceless consonant.

4. The mid-central lax vowel (unrounded/ unstressed)

5. "Duh!"

6. /ɚ/

7. Stressed syllables.

Chapter 12

1. /ɑ/

2. Lips round or slightly protrude.

3. Upsilon.

4. /ʊ/u/o/

5. bushel crook wolves put

Chapter 13

1. Two vowels spoken in sequence (in continuation).

2. There is a gradual movement of the articulators from one vowel to another.

3. ‿ To indicate two vowel sounds in each diphthongs are used together.

4. /aɪ/ /aʊ/ /ɔɪ/

5. /ju/

6. /aɪ/

Chapter 14

1. Accent.

2. Most prominent part of a syllable in a multisyllabic word or word in a phrase.

3. Stress placed on first or second syllable. For example: **sus**pect (noun: someone *suspected* of something) and sus**pect** (verb: believe someone is *guilty* of something).

4. Majority of morphological markers do not change stress in a word. The stress is usually on the root word and first syllable of a two-syllable word.

5. Words of two syllables have the same amount of stress. Example: textbook.

6. Stress has been associated with: (a) high amplitude (loudness), (b) long duration of the syllable nucleus (time), and (c) high frequency (pitch) of the syllable nucleus.

Chapter 15

1. Adjustment or adaptation of speech sounds due to phonetic environment.

2. Phonemes which surround a specific speech sound.

3. Assimilation and co-articulation.

4. Progressive: Occurs left to right. A *preceding* phoneme influences the phoneme.
   Regressive: Occurs right to left. A phoneme is changed by one that *follows* it.

5. Occurs as a result of the rapid rate of speech. Produces minor phonetic changes.

6. A symbol to indicate a specific way a phoneme was produced.

7. Lengthening diacritic is ː or ˑ

8. When a voiced phoneme is adjacent to an unvoiced phoneme. Example: price [praɪs]

9. Elision: A phoneme is omitted in a word. Example: "cam-er-a" [kæmrə]
   Epenthesis: Phoneme can be added. Example: "spoon" [səpun]

Chapter 16

1. Accent-free speech.

2. A variation of speech or language.

3. Speech characteristics of a foreign dialect.

4. East, Midwest, Southern states.

5. /t/ substitution for /θ/ in Initial position; consonant cluster reduction; /r/ phoneme lessened or omitted.

6. b/v substitution, schwa inserted before Initial consonant clusters, Spanish "s" produced frontally.

Table of Contents for CDs

CD 1—Transcription Exercises

Track	Exercise	Description	Page	Track	Exercise	Description	Page
1	—	Intro to CDs	—	37	TE 6–9	Fricatives /s/z/f/v/	105
2	TE 2–1	Sounds in Words	15	38	TE 6–10	/θ/	106
3	TE 2–2	Phoneme Fill In	16	39	TE 6–11	/θ/	107
4	TE 2–3	Phoneme Identification	17	40	TE 6–12	/ð/	109
5	TE 4–1	/p/	40	41	TE 6–13	/ð/	110
6	TE 4–2	/p/	41	42	TE 6–14	Listening for /θ/ð/	112
7	TE 4–3	/b/	43	43	TE 6–15	Fricatives: /θ/ð/	115
8	TE 4–4	/b/	44	44	TE 6–16	/h /	116
9	TE 4–5	/t/	48	45	TE 6–17	/h/	117
10	TE 4–6	/t/	49	46	TE 6–18	/hw/ or /ʍ/	119
11	TE 4–7	Glottal Stop	51	47	TE 6–19	/hw/ or /ʍ/	120
12	TE 4–8	Voiced /t/	52	48	TE 6–20	/h/ /hw/ or /ʍ/	122
13	TE 4–9	/d/	54	49	TE 6–21	/ʃ/	123
14	TE 4–10	/d/	55	50	TE 6–22	/ʃ/	124
15	TE 4–11	/k/	58	51	TE 6–23	/ʒ/	126
16	TE 4–12	/k/	59	52	TE 6–24	/ʒ/	127
17	TE 4–13	/g/	61	53	TE 7–1	/tʃ/	134
18	TE 4–14	/g/	62	54	TE 7–2	/tʃ/	135
19	TE 4–15	Stop Consonants	66	55	TE 7–3	/dʒ/	137
20	TE 5–1	/m/	70	56	TE 7–4	/dʒ/	138
21	TE 5–2	/m/	71	57	TE 7–5	Fricatives and Affricates	142
22	TE 5–3	/n/	73	58	TE 8–1	/w/	146
23	TE 5–4	/n/	74	59	TE 8–2	/w/	147
24	TE 5–5	/ŋ/	77	60	TE 8–3	/j/	150
25	TE 5–6	/ŋ/	78	61	TE 8–4	/j/	151
26	TE 5–7	Nasal Consonants	84	62	TE 8–5	/l/	153
27	TE 5–8	Syllabics	85	63	TE 8–6	/l/	154
28	TE 6–1	/f/	88	64	TE 8–7	/r/	156
29	TE 6–2	/f/	89	65	TE 8–8	/r/	157
30	TE 6–3	/v/	91	66	TE 8–9	/ir/	160
31	TE 6–4	/v/	92	67	TE 8–10	/ɛr/	161
32	TE 6–5	/s/	96	68	TE 8–11	/ɑr/	162
33	TE 6–6	/s/	97	69	TE 8–12	/or/	163
34	TE 6–7	/z/	99	70	TE 8–13	Vowel + /r/	167
35	TE 6–8	/z/	100	71	TE 8–14	Oral Resonant Consonants	168
36	Listening Exercise	Listening for /z/	102				

CD 2—Transcription Exercises

CD 3—Study Card Tracks

Study Card #	Phoneme	Track	Study Card #	Phoneme	Track
1	/k/	1	25	/w/	25
2	/g/	2	26	/i/	26
3	/p/	3	27	/ɪ/	27
4	/b/	4	28	/ɛ/	28
5	/t/	5	29	/e/	29
6	/d/	6	30	/æ/	30
7	/s/	7	31	/ə/	31
8	/z/	8	32	/ʌ/	32
9	/f/	9	33	/ɚ/	33
10	/v/	10	34	/ɝ/	34
11	/θ/	11	35	/u/	35
12	/ð/	12	36	/ʊ/	36
13	/ʃ/	13	37	/o/	37
14	/ʒ/	14	38	/ɔ/	38
15	/h/	15	39	/ɑ/	39
16	/hw/	16	40	/aɪ/	40
17	/tʃ/	17	41	/aʊ/	41
18	/dʒ/	18	42	/ɔɪ/	42
19	/m/	19	43	/ju/	43
20	/n/	20	44	/ɑr/	44
21	/ŋ/	21	45	/or/	45
22	/l/	22	46	/ir/	46
23	/j/	23	47	/ɛr/	47
24	/r/	24			

References

Battle, D. E. (Ed.). (2012). *Communicative disorders in multicultural and international populations* (4th ed.). St Louis, MO: Elsevier.

Bernthal, J., & Bankson, N. (1998). Phonological assessment procedures. In *Articulation and phonological disorders* (4th ed.). Boston, MA: Allyn & Bacon.

Edwards, H. T. (2003). *Applied phonetics: The sounds of American English* (3rd ed.). Clifton Park, NY: Thomson Delmar Learning.

Garn-Nunn, P., & Lynn, J. (2004). *Calvert's descriptive phonetics* (3rd ed.). New York, NY: Thieme.

Hegde, M. N. & Pomaville, F. (2013). *Assessment of communicative disorders in children* (2nd ed.). San Diego, CA: Plural.

Ladefoged, P. (2005). *Vowels and consonants* (2nd ed.). Malden, MA: Blackwell.

Lowe, R. J. & Blosser, J. (2002). *Workbook for identification of phonological processes and distinctive features* (4th ed.). Austin, TX: Pro-Ed.

MacKay, I. (1987). *Phonetics: The science of speech production* (2nd ed.) Boston, MA: Allyn & Bacon.

Mann, W. (2012). *Hello, gorgeous: Becoming Barbra Streisand.* Boston, MA: Houghton Mifflin Harcourt.

McLaughlin, S. (2006). *Introduction to language development* (2nd ed.) Clifton Park, NY: Thomson Delmar Learning.

Pena-Brooks, A., & Hegde, M. N. (2007). *Assessment and treatment of phonological disorders in children.* Austin, TX: Pro-Ed.

Roseberry-McKibbin, C. (2002). *Multicultural students with special needs: Practical strategies for assessment and intervention.* Oceanside, CA: Academic Communication Associates.

Shipley, K., & McAfee, J. G. (2008). *Assessment in speech-language pathology* (4th ed.). Clifton Park, NY: Delmar Cengage Learning.

Shriberg, L., & Kent, R. D. (2012). *Clinical phonetics* (4th ed.). Boston, MA: Pearson.

Singh, S., & Singh, K. (2006). *Phonetics: Principles and practices* (3rd ed.). San Diego, CA: Plural.

Glossary

abduction   movement of vocal folds to open the space between the folds; folds do not vibrate

adduction   movement of vocal folds to close the space between the folds; folds vibrate

affricate   phonemes that begin with a stop consonant and end with production of a fricative, e.g., /tʃ/ and /dʒ/

African American English   a dialect of English

alveolar ridge   structure located behind upper teeth; also known as the gum ridge

approximation   a position of closeness of the articulators that causes some constriction; associated with oral resonant consonants

articulation   modification of the breath stream by organs of the speech mechanism to produce speech

aspiration   release of impounded air for production of a stop-consonant

assimilation   a type of accommodation; produces major changes that occur when a phoneme is omitted, added, or changed to a different phoneme

bilabial   phonemes produced by contact of both lips, e.g., /b/

bound morpheme   a morpheme that must be bound to another morpheme to convey meaning, e.g., *cats*

broad transcription   transcription of sounds using IPA; no diacritics used

closed syllable   a syllable that contains a consonant in the final position

coarticulation   a type of accommodation; produces minor changes in phonemes

coda   consonant(s) that appear after a vowel in a syllable; not all syllables contain a coda

cognate   phonemes made in the same place and manner of articulation; only voicing differs

consonant   sound produced with a complete or partially obstructed vocal tract

cluster   two or more adjacent consonants in the same syllable, e.g., *spring, blue, fast*

dentals referring to the teeth

diacritic symbol indicating a specific way a phoneme has been produced

diphthong two vowels spoken in continuation; an onglide or offglide

distinctive features system describing attributes of a phoneme required to differentiate one phoneme from another, e.g., distinguishing feature of /k/ and /g/ is voicing

elision omission of a phoneme in a word or phrase

epenthesis addition of a phoneme

epiglottis a structure that acts like a cover for the opening to the larynx to prevent food and drink from entering trachea

free morpheme morpheme that can stand alone to convey meaning, e.g., *cat*

fricative consonants produced with partial blockage of the airstream, resulting in turbulence or friction

glide a consonant produced with relatively unobstructed vocal tract such as /w/j/r/

glottal referring to the glottis

glottal stop speech sound produced when vocal folds partially adduct to create buildup of air pressure; written as ?

glottis space between the vocal folds

hard palate anterior 2/3 of roof of the mouth, separates oral and nasal cavities

homorganic sounds produced in the same place and manner; /ŋ/ and /k/ and /g/ are homorganic

IPA International Phonetic Alphabet; specialized sound-symbol system that represents sounds of languages

intervocalic consonant located between two vowels, e.g., cookie

labial referring to the lips

labiodental consonant produced with lower lip and upper central incisors, e.g., /f/ and /v/

larynx structure composed of cartilage and muscles; vocal folds are located in the larynx

lateral sound produced with airstream directed around the sides of the tongue, e.g., /l/

lax vowel produced with reduced muscular effort

lingua referring to the tongue; Latin for "tongue"

lingual frenum small, white cord of tissue located on floor of oral cavity to midline of under surface of tongue blade

liquid generic term for /r/ and /l/ consonants

lungs respiratory organ that provides a breath stream for speech

mandible lower jaw

maxilla upper jaw

monophthong single vowel sound

morpheme minimal meaningful unit of language

narrow transcription transcription of speech sounds that uses diacritics to indicate specific way a sound is produced

nucleus part of the composition of a syllable, usually a vowel

obstruent consonant produced with full or partial blockage of the vocal tract

offglide movement of tongue from lower to higher vowel (movement from vowel of longer duration to one of shorter duration) in diphthong production, e.g., /aʊ/

onglide diphthong movement from a preceding sound into a vowel of longer duration, e.g., /ju/

onset consonant that precedes a vowel in a syllable, e.g., *dog*; not all syllables contain an onset

open syllable syllable containing a vowel in final position, e.g., *go*

palatal consonants produced by body of tongue contacting or approximating the posterior portion of the hard palate, e.g., /ʃ/ʒ/tʃ/dʒ/j/

PARR reference to speech as end product of four processes of *Phonation, Articulation, Respiration and, Resonation*

pharynx tubular-shaped structure; serves as a resonating tract

phonation adduction of vocal folds for voiced sounds

phoneme speech sound that can be distinguished from other speech sounds

place of articulation location of specific articulators used in production of a specific phoneme

postvocalic consonant consonant that follows a vowel

prevocalic consonant consonant that precedes a vowel

progressive assimilation preceding phoneme influences a phoneme that follows; occurs left to right in an utterance

respiration flow of air from lungs; exhaled air is used for speech

resonance process of vibrating air in a resonating cavity, e.g., oral or nasal cavity

rhyme part of a syllable consisting of a nucleus and optional coda

SAE (*Standard American English*) form of English that is "accent free"

sibilant consonant produced with a "hissing" sound such as /s/ or /ʃ/

sonorants consonant produced by a relatively open vocal tract

stop consonant consonant produced with complete obstruction of the airstream

syllabic consonant consonant with a vowel-like quality

tap also called "flap." Manner of production of consonant that is a rapid tongue movement against the alveolar ridge, i.e., /ɾ/

tense description of vowel produced by increased muscular effort

tongue advancement used in the vowel quadrangle; refers to how far forward in the oral cavity the tongue is located; horizontal dimension of the VQ

tongue height used in the vowel quadrangle; refers to tongue height in the vertical dimension of the VQ

trachea cartilaginous tube composed of rings; connects larynx with lungs

transcription   using IPA symbols to represent speech sounds

velar   consonants produced when back portion of tongue contacts velum, e.g., /k/g/ŋ/

velopharyngeal valve   composed of the velum and musculature of the posterior pharyngeal wall

velum   soft palate located posterior to the hard palate

vocal folds   folds of elastic tissue composed of muscles

voiced   phoneme produced with vocal fold vibration

voiceless   phoneme produced without vocal fold vibration

vowel   phoneme produced with relatively open vocal tract

vowel quadrangle (VQ)   figure representing production of vowels with reference to tongue height and advancement in the oral cavity

Index

Phoneme Study Cards

#1
Voiceless Lingua-Velar Stop-Consonant /k/

Initial	cab	[kæb]
Medial	acorn	[ekorn]
Final	fake	[fek]

#2
Voiced Lingua-Velar Stop-Consonant /g/

Initial	game	[gem]
Medial	begin	[biˈgɪn]
Final	mug	[mʌg]

#3
Voiceless Bilabial Stop-Consonant /p/

Initial	paid	[ped]
Medial	repeat	[riˈpit]
Final	lamp	[læmp]

#4
Voiced Bilabial Stop-Consonant /b/

Initial	burn	[bɝn]
Medial	habit	[ˈhæbɪt]
Final	probe	[prob]

#5
Voiceless Lingua-Alveolar Stop-Consonant /t/

Initial	tea	[ti]
Medial	material	[məˈtɪriəl]
Final	cot	[kɑt]

#6
Voiced Lingua-Alveolar Stop-Consonant /d/

Initial	drop	[drɑp]
Medial	radar	[redar]
Final	yard	[jard]

#7
Voiceless Lingua-Alveolar Fricative /s/

Initial	same	[sem]
Medial	missing	[ˈmɪsɪŋ]
Final	cuffs	[kʌfs]

#8
Voiced Lingua-Alveolar Fricative /z/

Initial	zone	[zon]
Medial	pansy	[ˈpænzi]
Final	clams	[klæmz]

#9
Voiceless Labiodental Fricative /f/

Initial	fern	[fɝn]
Medial	coffee	[ˈkafi]
Final	wife	[waɪf]

f

z

s

p

t

b

p

g

k

#10
Voiced Labiodental Fricative /v/

Initial	verb	[vɝb]
Medial	envy	[ɛnvi]
Final	eve	[iv]

#11
Voiceless Interdental Fricative /θ/

Initial	thick	[θɪk]
Medial	toothpaste	['tuθpest]
Final	booth	[buθ]

#12
Voiced Interdental Fricative /ð/

Initial	then	[ðɛn]
Medial	gather	[gæˈðɚ]
Final	bathe	[beð]

#13
Voiceless Lingua-Palatal Fricative /ʃ/

Initial	shake	[ʃek]
Medial	fishing	['fɪʃɪŋ]
Final	rush	[rʌʃ]

#14
Voiced Lingua-Palatal Fricative /ʒ/

Initial	Does not exist in SAE	
Medial	leisure	['liʒɚ]
Final	beige	[beʒ]

#15
Voiceless Glottal Fricative /h/

Initial	ham	[hæm]
Medial	inhale	[ɪnhel]
Final	Does not exist in SAE	

#16
Voiceless Labial-Velar Fricative /hw/

Initial	whirl	[hwɝəl]
Medial	buckwheat	[bʌkhwit]
Final	Does not exist in isolation in SAE	

#17
Voiceless Alveopalatal Affricate /tʃ/

Initial	chirp	[tʃɝp]
Medial	future	['fjutʃɚ]
Final	research	[riˈsɝtʃ]

#18
Voiced Alveopalatal Affricate /dʒ/

Initial	gel	[dʒɛl]
Medial	magic	[mædʒɪk]
Final	package	[pækɪdʒ]

dʒ tʃ hw

h ʒ ʃ

ɚ θ ʌ

#19
Voiced Bilabial Nasal /m/

Initial — marsh — [marʃ]
Medial — comedy — [kamɛdi]
Final — alarm — [ʌlaɾm]

#20
Voiced Lingua-Alveolar Nasal /n/

Initial — near — [nir]
Medial — canal — [kʌnæl]
Final — pelican — [pɛlɪkɪn]

#21
Voiced Velar Nasal /ŋ/

Initial — Does not exist in SAE
Medial — finger — [fɪŋgɚ]
Final — asking — [æskɪŋ]

#22
Voiced Lingua-Alveolar Lateral Liquid /l/

Initial — leaf — [lif]
Medial — dollar — [dɑlɚ]
Final — scandal — [skændəl]

#23
Voiced Lingua-Palatal On-Glide /j/

Initial — yogurt — [jogɚt]
Medial — kayak — [kajæk]
Final — Does not exist in SAE

#24
Voiced Alveo-Palatal Liquid (Glide) /r/

Initial — raid — [red]
Medial — fabric — [fæbrɪk]
Final — car — [kar]

#25
Voiced Bilabial (Lingua-Velar) Glide /w/

Initial — west — [wɛst]
Medial — reward — [riword]
Final — Does not exist in SAE

#26
High Front Tense Unrounded Vowel /i/

Initial — east — [ist]
Medial — beef — [bif]
Final — me — [mi]

#27
High Front Lax Unrounded Vowel /ɪ/

Initial — in — [ɪn]
Medial — finish — [fɪnɪʃ]
Final — city — [sɪtɪ]

Note: The /ɪ/ in SAE occurs in words ending in "y."

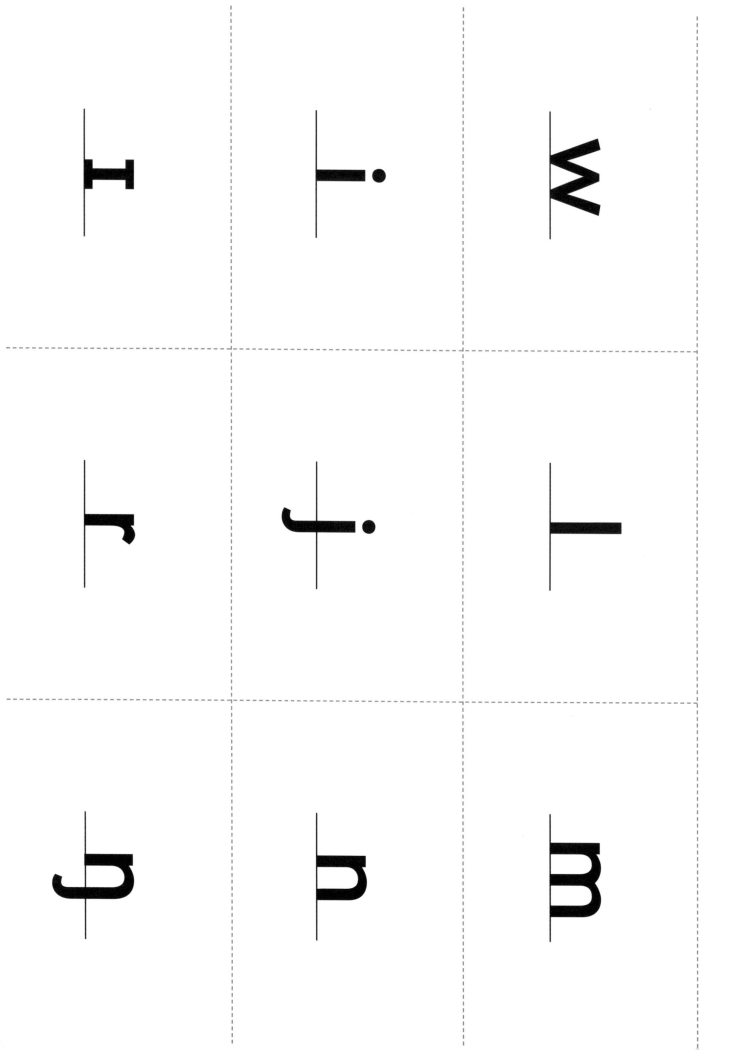

#34
Mid-Central R-Colored Tense Vowel (Stressed) /ɝ/

Initial	irk	[ɝk]
Medial	turn	[tɝn]
Final	purr	[pɝ]

#35
High Back Tense Rounded Vowel /u/

Note: /u/ rarely occurs in initial position in SAE, such as in "oops."

Medial	boom	[bum]
Final	chew	[tʃu]

#36
High Back Lax Rounded Vowel /ʊ/

Does not occur in initial or final positions of words in SAE.

Medial	hook	[hʊk]
	butcher	[ˈbʊtʃɚ]

#31
Mid-Central Lax Unrounded Vowel (Unstressed) (Schwa) /ə/

Initial	amuse	[əˈmjuz]
Medial	ravine	[rəvin]
Final	sofa	[sofə]

#32
Mid-Central Unrounded Vowel (Stressed) /ʌ/

Initial	oven	[ʌvin]
Medial	bumpy	[ˈbʌmpl]
Final	Does not exist in SAE	

#33
Mid-Central R-Colored Lax Vowel (Unstressed) /ɚ/

Initial	urbane	[ɚˈben]
Medial	scattering	[skætɚɪŋ]
Final	mayor	[mejɚ]

#28
Mid Front Lax Unrounded Vowel /ɛ/

Initial	echo	[ɛko]
Medial	dent	[dɛnt]
Final	Does not exist in SAE	

#29
Mid-Front Tense Unrounded Vowel /e/

Initial	aim	[em]
Medial	bake	[bek]
Final	way	[we]

#30
Low Front Lax Unrounded Vowel /æ/

Initial	at	[æt]
Medial	hatrack	[ˈhætræk]
Final	Does not exist in SAE	

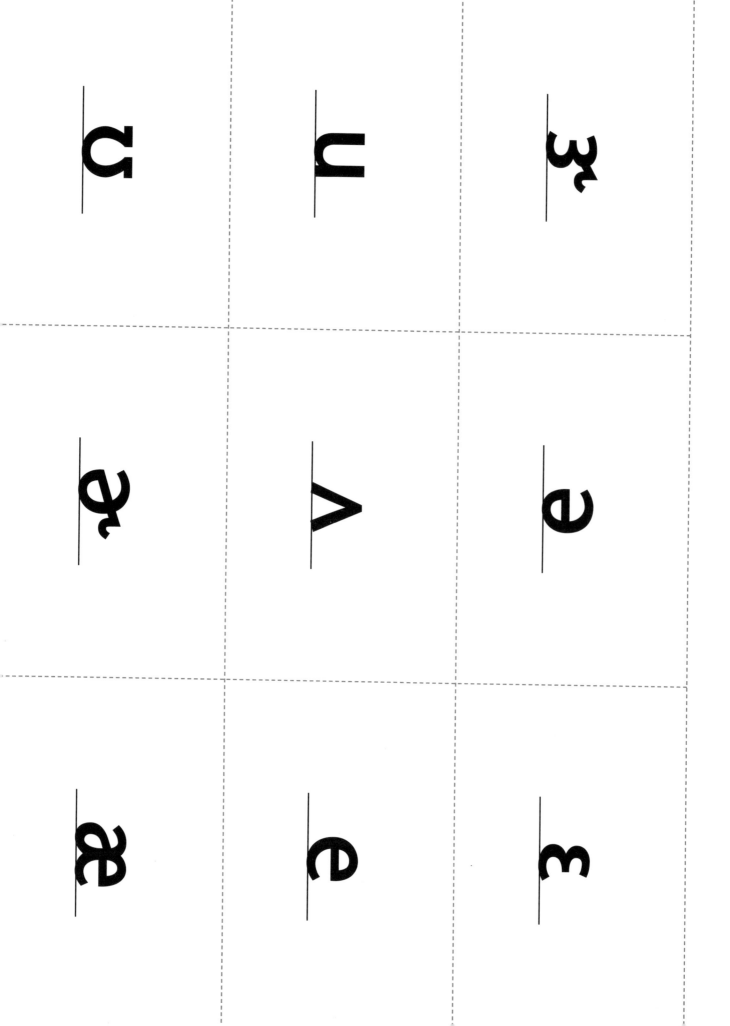

#37
Mid-Back Tense Rounded Vowel /o/

Initial	open	[ˈopɪn]
Medial	pole	[pol]
Final	sew	[so]

#38
Low Mid-Back Lax Rounded Vowel /ɔ/

Initial	ostrich	[ˈɔstrɪtʃ]
Medial	dawn	[dɔn]
Final	thaw	[θɔ]

#39
Low Back Lax Unrounded Vowel /ɑ/

Initial	encore	[ankor]
Medial	calm	[kɑlm]
Final	spa	[spɑ]

#40
Rising Low Front to High Front (Off-Glide) Diphthong /aɪ/

Initial	eye	[aɪ]
Medial	pine	[paɪn]
Final	sigh	[saɪ]

#41
Rising Low Front to High Back (Off-Glide) Diphthong /aʊ/

Initial	ouch	[aʊtʃ]
Medial	brown	[braʊn]
Final	vow	[vaʊ]

#42
Rising Mid-Back to High Front (Off-Glide) Diphthong /ɔɪ/

Initial	oil	[ɔɪl]
Medial	join	[dʒɔɪn]
Final	deploy	[dɪplɔɪ]

#43
High Front to High Back (On-Glide) Diphthong /ju/

Initial	use	[juz]
Medial	huge	[hjudʒ]
Final	pew	[pju]

j͡u

ɔ͡ɪ   a͡ʊ   a͡ɪ

ɑ   ɔ   o

#44
Vowel + r sequence /ɑr/

Initial	*ark*	[ɑrk]
Medial	*garden*	[gɑrdɪn]
Final	*star*	[stɑr]

#45
Vowel + r sequence /or/

Initial	*oar*	[or]
Medial	*norm*	[norm]
Final	*your*	[jor]

#46
Vowel + r sequence /ir/

Initial	*era*	[irʌ]
Medial	*fierce*	[firs]
Final	*here*	[hir]

#47
Vowel + r sequence /ɛr/

Initial	*error*	[ɛrɚ]
Medial	*perish*	[ˈpɛrɪʃ]
Final	*stare*	[stɛr]

er

or

3r

ar